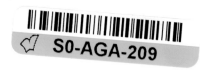

TECHNIQUES
OF
PATIENT-ORIENTED
RESEARCH

TECHNIQUES
OF
PATIENT-ORIENTED
RESEARCH

Editors

CHARLES Y.C. PAK, M.D.
Distinguished Chair in Mineral Metabolism
University of Texas Southwestern Medical Center
Dallas, Texas

PERRIE M. ADAMS, Ph.D.
Associate Dean
University of Texas Southwestern Medical Center
Dallas, Texas

Raven Press New York

Raven Press, Ltd., 1185 Avenue of the Americas, New York, New York 10036

Made in the United States of America

Library of Congress Cataloging-in-Publication Data

Techniques of patient-oriented research/edited by Charles Y.C. Pak.
    Perrie M. Adams.
        p.   cm.
    Includes bibliographical references and index.
    ISBN 0-7817-0107-4
    1. Clinical trials.   2. Medicine—Research—Methodology.   I. Pak,
Charles Y.C.   II. Adams, Perrie M.
    [DNLM: 1. Research Design.   W 20.5 T255 1993]
RC853.C55T43   1994
610'.72—dc20
DNLM/DLC
For Library of Congress   93-4602
                                                                CIP

9 8 7 6 5 4 3 2 1

Contents

CONTENTS

Contributing Authors

Perrie M. Adams, Ph.D.   Associate Dean for Research, University of Texas Southwestern Medical Center at Dallas, 5323 Harry Hines Blvd., Dallas, Texas 75235-8885

Neil A. Breslau, M.D.   Program Director, GCRC, Professor of Medicine, University of Texas Southwestern Medical Center at Dallas, 5323 Harry Hines Blvd., Dallas, Texas 75235-8885

Linda Brinkley, R.D.   Research Dietitian, GCRC, University of Texas Southwestern Medical Center at Dallas, 5323 Harry Hines Blvd., Dallas, Texas 75235-8885

Katherine L. Chapman, J.D.   Associate Vice-President for Legal Affairs and Technology Transfer, University of Texas Southwestern Medical Center at Dallas, 5323 Harry Hines Blvd., Dallas, Texas 75235-8885

Scott M. Grundy, M.D., Ph.D.   Director, Center for Human Nutrition, Professor of Medicine, University of Texas Southwestern Medical Center at Dallas, 5323 Harry Hines Blvd., Dallas, Texas 75235-8885

Robert W. Haley, M.D.   Chief, Epidemiology Division, Associate Professor of Medicine, University of Texas Southwestern Medical Center at Dallas, 5323 Harry Hines Blvd., Dallas, Texas 75235-8885

Charles Y.C. Pak, M.D.   Assistant Dean for Clinical Research and Distinguished Chair in Mineral Metabolism, University of Texas Southwestern Medical Center at Dallas, 5323 Harry Hines Blvd., Dallas, Texas 75235-8885

CONTRIBUTING AUTHORS

Joan S. Reisch, Ph.D. Biostatistician and Director of Academic Computing Services, University of Texas Southwestern Medical Center at Dallas, 5323 Harry Hines Blvd., Dallas, Texas 75235-8885

Joseph E. Zerwekh, Ph.D. Professor of Medicine, University of Texas Southwestern Medical Center at Dallas, 5323 Harry Hines Blvd., Dallas, Texas 75235-8885

Preface

The explosive advances in molecular medicine have revolution-ized basic approaches in biomedical research. Unfortunately, clinical research has lagged because of a worker shortage and insufficient funding. This widening gap could erode the transla-tion of discoveries in the laboratory to the patient.

A major factor for the slowdown in clinical research, though not the sole one, is inadequate training. The medical school curricu-lum is usually lacking in rigorous training programs in instruction of techniques in clinical research. The relatively poor showing of clinical research grants may be partly due to poor preparation of grant applications and inadequate training of clinical investiga-tors, rather than to poor science.

Detailed training in clinical research depends on the type of clinical research and the level of clinical investigators. However, anyone interested in performing clinical research at whatever type or level needs to be aware of the basic principles of clinical research, the latest regulatory guidelines, and the available resources. This book is designed to meet that need.

Different categories of clinical research are compared, and the need for clinical research training is described in Chapter 1. Conflict of interest that might arise during the course of clinical research are addressed in Chapter 2. Chapters 3 and 4 describe updated guidelines on informed consent, protocol preparation, and research grant applications. Various study designs and appropriate statistical approaches are introduced in Chapters 5 and 6. Chapter 7 details various general laboratory techniques utilized in clinical research. In Chapter 8 the role of nutrition in clinical research is considered from the perspective of supporting metabolic studies and pursuing primary nutritional research questions. Resources of general clinical research centers in carrying out patient-oriented research are described in Chapter

PREFACE

9, and finally, elements of manuscript preparation are presented in Chapter 10.

Charles Y.C. Pak
Perrie M. Adams

Acknowledgment

This book is based on successful seminars on the introduction and practice of patient-oriented research held at the University of Texas Southwestern Medical School over the past several years. The authors are the senior faculty members who participated in the seminars as lecturers. We humbly acknowledge their enthusiasm, dedication, and commitment. Without them, the publication of this book would not have been possible.

TECHNIQUES
OF
PATIENT-ORIENTED
RESEARCH

1

Clinical Research in the 1990s

Problems and Challenges

Charles Y. C. Pak

Center for Mineral Metabolism and Clinical Research, University of Texas Southwestern Medical Center at Dallas, Dallas, Texas 75235-8885

Clinical research in the 1990s is at an important crossroads, facing many problems and challenges. Exciting advances in the laboratory, particularly in molecular biology, have given clinical researchers unparalleled opportunities for research, but our ability to meet these challenges is continually being eroded.

THE ATTRITION OF YOUNG CLINICAL INVESTIGATORS

A major problem is the attrition of young clinical investigators. We are faced with a realistic possibility that there may not be a sufficient number of trained clinical investigators to translate basic knowledge obtained from laboratory investigation to the patient's bedside. There are surely other pressing problems

1

facing clinical research in the 1990s, such as the challenges of the continuing epidemic of the acquired immunodeficiency syndrome (AIDS) and those of gene therapy. However, the problem of attrition of young clinical investigators is critical; if not corrected, this attrition could severely curtail clinical research even if its other problems are resolved.

We have all observed and suffered from the attrition of young clinical investigators. An increasing number of promising clinical researchers have left us for industry or for private practice. Fewer young physicians are choosing a career in academic medicine.

In 1977, Dr. S. O. Thier, in his presidential address to the American Federation for Clinical Research, noted that the percentage of medical school faculty younger than 40 years declined from 47% in 1967 to 27% in 1977 (3). The percentage of National Institutes of Health (NIH) grant applications by investigators less than 36 years of age declined from 25.4% in 1980 to 15.5% in 1990 (1). No wonder that Dr. Thier declared: "The endangered species today is . . . the M.D.-investigator."

Why is there attrition of young clinical investigators? First, restricted research funding, particularly from the NIH, has severely curtailed the ability of young investigators to mount independent research and has often subjugated them to sponsor parochialism or servitude. Second, increased federal and state guidelines for clinical research have necessitated the expenditure of seemingly useless effort in paperwork, leaving less time for research. Third, dramatic advances in basic research have made clinical research less attractive. It is my firm conviction that basic and clinical research are complementary. Discoveries in the laboratory require translation into clinical practice. In the setting of the general clinical research center (GCRC), there is still ample room for well-controlled metabolic studies that do not require molecular biology. Yet recent exciting advances in the laboratory have led to the disparagement of clinical research at various sectors. The NIH R01 applications (research grants submitted by individuals) that use molecular biological techniques in pursuit of a clinical objective seem to be better received than grants that do not. At many institutions, M.D. molecular biologists are more likely to be given tenure than are clinical researchers.

The NIH's own figures support reduced research funding. The NIH's share of health-related research progressively decreased from 40% of total health-related awards in 1980 to 32% in 1990 (2). Despite a large increase in the number of research grant applications received by the NIH during the past 10 years, the actual number of funded grants remained relatively constant.

The funding has been particularly precarious for clinical research. The percentage of new R01 applications submitted by M.D.s declined from 27.2%

TABLE 1. *Topics for discussion*

Definition of clinical research
Implementation of training program
Personal commitment and dedication

in 1980 to 25.4% in 1990; the remaining 74.6% were submitted by Ph.D.s. Only 28.8% of grants submitted by M.D.s were funded in 1990 (1).

I recently served as a member of a committee to examine the state of clinical research funding. There were ten NIH intramural and ten extramural scientists. The committee was called INEX to reflect intramural and extramural participation. We randomly selected approximately 200 of about 2,000 funded R01 applications during index years—1977, 1982, and 1987. The members of the INEX committee personally reviewed selected funded grants and identified those that dealt with intense research in whole human beings. Such patient-oriented research projects comprised 7.8% of funded grants in 1977, 8.1% in 1982, and a paltry 6.0% in 1987.

With the above background, I will address three topics for discussion (Table 1). I will define clinical research and share with you my thoughts for the implementation of training programs for young clinical researchers. I will then make a plea to all of you for personal commitment and dedication to clinical research.

My underlying assumptions are that (a) there is a need for training of investigators at all categories of clinical research, (b) many clinical researchers are poorly trained and inadequately equipped to compete effectively for research grants and to apply discoveries in basic sciences to the patient's bedside, (c) improved training and support of young clinical investigators could stem the tide of attrition of young clinical investigators, and (d) important challenges and rewards await clinical researchers.

THE DEFINITION OF CLINICAL RESEARCH

Clinical research, in contrast to basic research, deals with human beings rather than experimental animals (Table 2). It is interested in the function of the whole human being instead of cells or molecules. Its approach is integrative rather than separative.

TABLE 2. *Definition of clinical research*

Human beings vs. experimental animals
Whole organisms vs. cells/molecules
Integrative vs. separative

There are several categories of clinical research (Table 3). Basic clinical research is the in-depth laboratory examination of specimens obtained from patients. It may be exemplified by the demonstration of defective low-density lipoprotein (LDL) receptor binding in patients with familial hypercholesterolemia. Patient-oriented research is represented by the physiological and metabolic exploration of human subjects, as is typically conducted at the GCRCs. It may be represented by differentiation of hypercalciuric nephrolithiasis into absorptive, renal, and resorptive forms. Remaining forms of clinical research are clinical trials, epidemiological studies, and clinical observations.

Clinical research is difficult because it is more complex than basic research and has bioethical constraints. Moreover, exact answers may be lacking, and controlled study may sometimes be difficult to conduct. But clinical research still requires scientific discipline and hypothesis testing.

THE IMPLEMENTATION OF TRAINING PROGRAMS

Despite an obvious need for training, rigorous training programs for clinical researchers are generally lacking. When we offered an introductory course in clinical research last year at Dallas, two-thirds of the participants were assistant professors or associate professors and there was even one full professor, although the course was intended for postdoctoral fellows and instructors. This

TABLE 3. *Categories of clinical research*

Basic clinical research
Patient-oriented research
Clinical trials
Epidemiology
Clinical observations

experience indicated a poor exposure to clinical research techniques even among the established faculty.

My NIH study section experience, which is shared by other reviewers, is revealing. Contrary to popular view, the Ph.D. study section members are generally more generous in their review of clinical grant applications than are the M.D. members. More likely reasons for the relatively poor showing of clinical research grant applications are the facts that (a) clinical grants are often inferior in preparation, though not necessarily in science, and (b) clinical investigators often seem to be inadequately trained.

It is therefore clear that clinical researchers must be better trained if they are to compete effectively for research grants, if they are to meet exciting challenges of the 1990s, and if they are to curtail the attrition of young clinical investigators. Training requirements must vary with different categories of clinical research. Thus, specific training programs must be developed for each category of research. Types of training programs might be an introductory course in clinical research techniques, a course in direct on-hand experience in clinical research techniques, physician scientist training programs at two levels, the GCRC Clinical Associate Physician program, and the M.D.-Ph.D. program. I will focus on the first two programs.

The Seminar on Introduction to Clinical Research as it is now offered at Dallas comprises ten 90-minute seminars that are held monthly, given by senior faculty, and cover the following topics: the definition of clinical research, conflict of interest and ethics, grantsmanship and protocol preparation, biotechnology development, study design, statistical analysis, laboratory techniques, nutritional support, the role of the GCRC, and the rewards of clinical research (Table 4).

The Practice of Clinical Research, offered to those who took the introductory course, is designed to give direct hands-on experience in protocol preparation and lay consent, the conduct of research, data analysis, the composition of a scientific paper, grantsmanship, the preparation of a manuscript, grant application, and conflict of interest (Table 5). Materials from already completed, successful clinical projects are utilized for hands-on training. For those who have completed both courses, seed money has been obtained to fund innovative, promising projects.

The first level of training programs for physician scientists might be a refinement of existing clinical postdoctoral fellowships, taking 2 to 3 years after residency. It would integrate all postdoctoral training programs at a given institution. There would be an advocacy group, represented by an advisory committee with members from different departments or disciplines and headed by a senior faculty member serving as the program director. There might be an association or organization of postdoctoral fellows with regularly held meetings

TABLE 4. *Introduction to clinical research*

Comprised of ten 90-min. seminars, held monthly, given by senior faculty

Topics

Definition	Laboratory techniques
Conflict of interest and ethics	Nutritional support
Grantsmanship and protocol preparation	Role of GCRC
Biotechnology development	Study design
Statistical analysis	Success stories

to foster exchange. Opportunities would be provided to take an elective in graduate curriculum in basic sciences and in training seminars.

The second level of training programs for physician scientists might be a further refinement of the fellowship program, requiring 4 years after residency. It would comprise all facets of Level 1, plus the following features. There would be didactic course work in basic sciences, and there might be research rotations in basic laboratories. The clinical load would be sufficient for the acquisition or maintenance of clinical skills but would not be overwhelming. As junior faculty members in the later years of this program, the physician scientists would be provided a salary adequate to avoid "moonlighting," and funds would be sought to help relieve debt incurred during their medical school training. They would be offered close support and guidance in research grant acquisition. Respective departments might be asked to help support this program, since it represents an investment in future productive members of the faculty.

I have not addressed the training of basic clinical researchers because I don't believe the need is as great. Besides M.D.-Ph.D. programs, there are many NIH training opportunities: K04 Research Career Development Awards, K08

TABLE 5. *Practice of clinical research*

Comprised of ten 90-min. seminars for those who took introductory course, designed to give direct on-hand experience

Topics

Introduction of research problem	Composition of scientific paper
Protocol and lay consent	Preparation of manuscript
Conduct of research	Grant application
Data analysis	Conflict of interest
Grantsmanship	

Clinical Investigator Awards, and K11 Physician Scientist Awards. In contrast to these existing opportunities, training needs that I am addressing are in clinical rather than in basic research, are institutionally based rather than individually acquired, and are directed at an earlier stage of development.

It is expected that various forms of the training programs described above would target different populations of young clinical scientists. Whatever the nature of training program adopted, it should be sufficiently diverse to equip researchers at all categories of clinical research. It should also be flexible so that an investigator at one level may learn to conduct clinical research at another level. Training programs should incorporate existing training mechanisms. Promising applicants should be encouraged to seek existing grant opportunities, such as K08 and K11 from the NIH; they could then be incorporated into system-wide training programs. The traditional training programs have been based on the tutor-student relationship. I am suggesting that current complexities of clinical research mandate a system-wide or institutionally based training, at least during the initial period of training.

The training seminars (Introduction and Practice) should be useful for clinical investigators at all levels. This conviction has led to the preparation of this book on the techniques of patient-oriented research. The book includes key topics from both seminars.

DEDICATION AND COMMITMENT TO CLINICAL RESEARCH

I plead with you to make a personal commitment and dedication to clinical research (Table 6). Unique challenges await M.D.s in clinical research. You can translate basic ideas into the understanding and treatment of human disease. You are the first to experience fruits of discoveries in the laboratory by testing them and assessing response in patients. You can also do the opposite, dissect human problems in the laboratory. Rewards are great. Besides the gratitude of patients and the potential for personal gratification, there is a greater chance that your work will improve patient care. To all clinical researchers among you, do not indulge in self-pity. Do not blame molecular biology for the plight of clinical

TABLE 6. *Challenges of MD's in clinical research*

Translation of basic ideas into understanding of human disease
Dissection of human problems in the laboratory
Potential for personal gratification and improved patient care delivery

TABLE 7. *Learn research techiniques*

Obtain an intimate knowledge of routine techniques
Get a working background in statistics and sophisticated methods
Never be afraid to take time out and to learn
Actively seek collaboration
Quality of research generally superior with unique research techniques

research. Rather, define your goals and become better equipped to compete more effectively for the dwindling dollar. I urge the seasoned clinical investigators among you to project a positive attitude, encourage young physicians to consider a career in clinical research, and advise them to seek adequate training to become better equipped to meet the challenges awaiting clinical research. To the young investigators among you, do not despair, look at the bright side, and consider the following suggestions.

Learn clinical research techniques (Table 7). Obtain intimate knowledge of routine techniques. Get a working background in statistics and sophisticated methods. Never be afraid to take time out to learn new techniques or approaches if needs arise. Be prepared to switch from one level of clinical research to another. Actively seek collaboration if you yourself don't possess or cannot learn essential techniques. Remember that the quality of research is generally superior the more unique the research technique. That particular research technique need not be molecular biology. It is any technique that is appropriate in solving the clinical problem at hand.

Recruit paramedical personnel in the conduct of your research. Involve nurses, dietitians, technicians, and statisticians as partners in research. Recognize their contribution as coauthors when appropriate. Increase their role from patient instruction and recruitment to protocol design and data analysis.

Try to accommodate limited research funding by learning research techniques, improving the quality of grant applications, and searching for alternate sources of funding (Table 8). If you fail, try and try again.

TABLE 8. *Accommodation of limited research funding*

Learn research techniques
Improve the quality of grants
Search for an alternative source of funding
Try and try again

TABLE 9. *Qualifications for a successful clinical researcher*

Be compassionate
Be imaginative but sensible
Work hard
Don't be easily discouraged
Be persistent

A radio evangelist in Dallas once espoused five Is to success in any walk of life: imagination, industry, initiative, integrity, and intelligence. They surely apply to clinical research as well.

I offer a slightly different version for the qualifications of a successful clinical researcher (Table 9). Be compassionate, as you are dealing with patients. Be imaginative but sensible. In other words, search constantly for new ideas for research but be discriminating. Work hard. Most importantly, don't be easily discouraged and be persistent. Reapply if your grants are not funded. If one idea fails, try another.

In closing, I want to remind you of that evening in August 1990 when Nolan Ryan obtained his 300th pitching win. In the bottom of the seventh inning, with Ryan's team ahead by 3 runs, the usually sure-handed teammate, second baseman Franco, made an error, allowing a run to come in for the opposing team. In the bottom of the eighth inning, Franco made another error, making the game closer and the win for Ryan precarious. You could see disgust in Franco's face as the television camera zoomed in on him. Then, in the top of the 9th, Franco came to bat with bases loaded. You could see determination in his face. He hit a grand-slam home run, assuring a history-making win for Ryan.

Like Franco, you should be persistent and should not be easily discouraged.

REFERENCES

1. Division of Research Grants, NIH (1980–1990): *DRG Peer Review Trends.* National Institutes of Health, Bethesda, MD.
2. National Institutes of Health (1991): *NIH Data Book.* NIH Publ. No. 91-1261. U.S. Department of Health and Human Services, Washington, DC.
3. Thier, S.O. (1977): Where do we go from here? An appeal to reason: AFCR Presidential Address, April 30. *Clin. Res.* 25:219–224.

2

Conflict of Interest

Katherine L. Chapman

Office of Legal Affairs, University of Texas Southwestern Medical Center at Dallas, Dallas, Texas 75235-9008

Clinical research has, perhaps more than any other category of health-related research, been influenced by the increased pharmaceutical industry funding in recent years. Although some basic research might go unfunded during a time of limited resources, clinical research cannot stop, since data are necessary to obtain legal approval of drugs for human use. Thus, as federal funding has declined, pharmaceutical industry funding of clinical research in the university setting has been expanding (2).

Concrete benefits of the industry-university association are clearly visible and have been for many years. In the late 1970s and the 1980s, even the federal government began, and it continues, to encourage and facilitate the translation of clinical research into practical medical products for the general public. Recognizing that university research has demonstrated the general economic value in marketing of products and processes, as well as improving the human condition, the mainstream thought has wholeheartedly approved the transfer of technology from the clinical researcher to the public. In the midst of this success, one cannot avoid also seeing the disadvantages of multifaceted industry-university association; if examined, the disadvantages can be openly dealt with in a way that will nurture the relationship and ultimately enhance health care.

Chief among these disadvantages is the potential for the existence or appearance of a conflict of interest or conflict of commitment which can obstruct the pathway of a needed drug, device, or process from the laboratory to the public. A loss of credibility in the eyes of society can result, so that no interests are served.

Issues of conflict of interest arise as a consequence of the antagonistic objectives of multitalented individuals. One does not desire success solely in one's field of research; one seeks success in other areas of life: civic, athletic, and, in this case, financial. In recent times personal economic gain from research has been acceptable so long as it has not resulted in a loss of scientific objectivity. However, in certain circumstances, that financial gain can open the door to a real conflict of interest or the appearance of one. The clinical investigator must be alert to events that may indicate the development of a conflict of interest or the appearance of one. Many articles address the obligations of the corporate entity; this chapter seeks to help the individual clinical investigator recognize the circumstances in which such conflicts may arise so that they can be avoided or mitigated.

THE DEFINITION OF CONFLICT OF INTEREST

Conflict of interest in clinical research means that personal, financial, or other interests may compromise, or appear to compromise, the professional responsibilities and standards of an investigator in carrying out or reporting clinical research. The compromising of an investigator's professional judgment may affect the choice of a project and methods; the gathering, analyzing, interpreting, and reporting of clinical data; the hiring of staff; and even purchasing (6). One author called clinical research that is open to conflict of interest "evaluative research—when an investigator acts on behalf of the public to test a new drug or device" (7). Such evaluative research is particularly susceptible to conflicts of interest and to the consequent loss of public confidence.

Conflicts of interest may be blatant or subtle, publicly known or privately guarded, visible or invisible. They differ from scientific misconduct or research fraud, such as falsification of data, plagiarism, or other such activities that discredit the integrity of one's research.

Regardless of the hue, conflicts of interest are insidious and must be discovered and dissipated by a clinical investigator to protect objectivity and hence one's data and scientific reputation. For example, the simplest of situations could cause a conflict of interest to arise: a clinical investigator owns a substantial number of shares of stock in a pharmaceutical company; the company financially sponsors the investigator's clinical research and will be the benefactor of research results; and the results favor the company's pharmaceutical product. Should the investigator not disclose this situation to the proper entities, an appearance, at best, and a true conflict, at worst, are likely to arise. Scientific careers have certainly been destroyed or at least irreparably tarnished by facts as simple as these. Some clinical investigators avoid such problems by choosing not to own stock or be financially tied to the company in any personal way that might appear to compromise the integrity of the investigator's research in violation of accepted standards of conduct. Others accept the personal benefits while relying on their good reputations to prevent an appearance of conflict. If successful, this may be seen as courageous. If unsuccessful, it will undoubtedly be viewed as foolhardy.

All investigators have standards of conduct or a code of ethics to which they must adhere. Some arise from employment; others from licensing bodies or guidelines of professional associations. These various standards of conduct are intended, in part, to increase public confidence in research institutions and clinical investigators and to solidify the researchers' priorities as well.

GUIDELINES FROM THE STATE OF TEXAS

Using Texas state-supported institutions of higher education within the University of Texas System as an example, we find a statutory conflict of interest provision, called "Standards of Conduct of State Officers and Employees" (11). It applies to all state employees, including, but not focused specifically on, faculty clinical investigators at state universities. For that reason, the comprehensive statement of standards of ethical conduct and conflicts of interest is general, although it can apply to the factual situations in which clinical investigators find themselves. The primary rule stated in this section is, "it is the policy of the State of Texas that no state officer or state employee shall have any interest, financial or otherwise, direct or indirect, or engage in any business transaction or professional activity or incur any obligation of any nature which is in substantial conflict with the proper discharge of his duties of the public interest" (11).

Substantial interest, which defines a substantial conflict presumably, is then defined in the statute as a controlling interest; ownership in excess of 10% of the voting interest in the business entity or in excess of $25,000 of the fair market value of the business entity; any participating interest, either direct or indirect, by shares, stock, or otherwise, whether or not voting rights are included, in the profits, proceeds, or capital gains of the business entity in excess of 10% of them; holding the position of a member of the board of directors or other governing board of the business entity; or being an employee of the business entity. The specific standards of conduct are spelled out in five detailed provisions, all of which begin, "No state . . . employee should . . . " (11). Again, however, one must be aware that these provisions apply to all state employees and not just state-employed faculty members, so that the prohibitions are very general.

OTHER GUIDELINES

Another example of the standards of conduct to which a clinical investigator may need to adhere comes from the American Federation for Clinical Research (AFCR). In this organization's Guidelines for Avoiding Conflict of Interest, the AFCR states that a potential conflict of interest is deemed to exist when an investigator appears to be in a position to receive a direct financial benefit from making positive observations and/or withholding negative information concerning a product under investigation. In these guidelines, *direct financial benefit* is not specifically defined. The examples described in the guidelines, however, would lead one to believe that it is not the amount of financial interest that concerns the AFCR. Rather, the AFCR is specifically concerned, as are others, with the appearance or reality of a company's fostering a personal relationship with the investigator (4). Accordingly, it is clear that, although some professional associations and university employers choose not to define personal financial gain specifically, others define it in great detail, as Texas does. Clinical investigators must know which statutes and guidelines apply specifically to them.

It might also be pointed out that many of the statutes, policies, and guidelines, such as the AFCR Guidelines (1), also apply to the family of the clinical investigator. Again, the extent to which the statute, policy, or guidelines extend to family members varies according to the particular entity setting forth the rules. Nevertheless, clinical investigators must recognize that, in many circumstances, anyone with whom they might have a familial connection may fall within the prohibitions, too. Putting stock ownership in the name of one's spouse or child will rarely dissipate a conflict of interest that exists between a clinical investigator and a business entity.

ARRANGEMENTS GENERATING CONFLICT OF INTEREST

There are many types of arrangements between clinical investigators and external entities that can result in the appearance or reality of a conflict of interest for the investigator. Some of them are noted here with an illustration of the kind of problem that might arise.

Clinical Trial Agreement

This type of agreement may be the most familiar to the clinical investigator. In its simplest form, a pharmaceutical company asks a clinical investigator to test its pharmaceutical product on a particular population (of patients and/or healthy individuals) to determine its effectiveness, correct dosage, and so forth. Receiving Food and Drug Administration approval of the drug will often be the company's goal. In other situations the pharmaceutical company may be supplying the drug at the investigator's behest to test the investigator's own hypothesis, which might ultimately benefit the company by giving the company more information about its drug. Funds may come to the investigator's employer to allow the investigator to perform the research. Sometimes offers to the clinical investigator of equity ownership in the company may be part of the arrangement, particularly if the company is small or a "start-up," as small companies are referred to in today's business vernacular. Many, if not most statutes, policies, and guidelines on conflict of interest would find that an investigator under the above fact situation who actually receives (or whose family actually receives) equity or the right to purchase shares of stock has a conflict of interest or, at the very best, the appearance of conflict of interest. This circumstance might well make the researcher subject to an allegation of bias in his or her research since the researcher could personally benefit from positive results of research on the company's drug.

Collaborative and Sponsored Research Agreements

Both collaborative and sponsored research agreements are also likely to produce the appearance of conflict of interest if the clinical investigator has ties to the industrial sponsor which could result in personal financial gain, since certain results could positively benefit the company sponsor or collaborator. In fact, in the current biotechnology marketplace, research findings reported by a business periodical one day can cause a fluctuation in price of the company's stock the next day. If the investigator owns stock or could realize personal benefit, it is not hard to see that questions regarding conflict of interest could arise.

Licenses

Patent or technology licenses are another way that conflict of interest issues can arise in the clinical investigator's career. If a clinical investigator is the inventor or developer of a new health-related product or process that is licensed by the investigator's employer to a commercial firm, a potential for conflict of interest arises when the inventor-investigator is offered equity or other personal financial benefits in exchange for the employer's rights to the product. The potential conflict may be dispelled by the fact that the investigator is not going to have any continuing relationship with the company-licensee or the product or process after the completion of a particular research study. The concern arises if the product or process is going to undergo subsequent testing or development by the same inventor-investigator, who will personally benefit from the marketing of the product. A continuing relationship between the investigator and the company selling the product may well lead to questions regarding the clinical investigator's ability to be objective in reporting results of the research on the drug.

Consulting Agreements

Consulting arrangements are ripe for conflict of interest problems. Many times investigators are asked to consult on general scientific issues with companies that are funding the clinical investigators' research. Although these arrangements could be innocent of conflicts of interest, an investigator should be aware of the possibilities, such as a claim that the investigator is receiving consulting funds or equity in such an amount that the researcher is guilty of bias. If the research is favorable to the company and the investigator personally benefits, the situation will surely be questioned.

There are other situations involving consulting agreements which might cause concern with regard to conflicts of interest. For example, if an investigator performed tests in his employer's facility and passed the results on to a company under a consulting arrangement, there would be an inappropriate use of institutional resources (i.e., to benefit the investigator personally). Depending on the employing entity, some investigators who are also physicians have different agreements with the employer regarding consulting. In some cases, the employer allows no external consulting in which the faculty member retains the funds personally.

Gifts

Pharmaceutical companies are historically known for presenting gifts to clinical investigators and their staffs, most often small tokens, such as scratch pads, umbrellas, or clocks. However, as noted before, the dollar value is not the issue. The fostering of a personal relationship between the physician and the company is the culprit (4) and may signal a conflict of interest. Clinical investigators and their staffs must be watchful to avoid the appearance of a conflict.

CONFLICT OF COMMITMENT

A less well-known type of conflict of interest should also concern clinical investigators. It is called *conflict of commitment* because it is theoretically based upon the clinical investigator's divided commitment of time: full-time to the employer and part-time to an outside third party, generally a pharmaceutical company. University-affiliated clinical investigators would not hesitate to recognize work for the university as "the primary and overriding obligation of every faculty member, in terms of his or her commitment of time, attention and intellectual energy"(8). However, they would also not hesitate to take the position that the university faculty member also has the right to time for consulting or working with commercial firms. One day a week is traditionally recognized as the allotment of time a faculty member can expect to be able to spend with a commercial or noncommercial firm without the conflict of commitment becoming a troublesome issue. While the rule may be written (5), it is just as often unwritten but followed.

The heart of each guideline on conflict of commitment, whether written or oral, is that the clinical investigator must acknowledge and behave in such a way that it is clear where the investigator's primary loyalty lies in terms of quantity and quality of research—that is, with the university.

THE CHARGE TO INVESTIGATORS

In dealing with any type of conflict of interest, most university employers have either written rules (such as Texas' statute mentioned above) or unwritten rules or customs to follow. The most common requirements of clinical investigators under conflict of interest rules and policies are (a) accountability and integrity and (b) disclosure of any potential conflicts of interest. Most universities have great trust in individuals' abilities to police themselves, and many policies reflect this through provisions for accountability. Disclosure of the potential conflict of interest by the individual involved is the other common requirement. Being sensitive to the situations that can bring an individual into a conflict of interest goes far in getting the individual off on the right foot with the employer. In fact, there are times that disclosure can be said to dispel the potential conflict. At other times, more severe action must be taken. Nevertheless, putting one's superiors on notice as soon as the potential for a conflict of interest is identified can favor the investigator tremendously in sorting out the various issues and making the decisions that must be made.

Grantors, or those who fund clinical research, whether federal, state, or private, may well have their own policies on conflict of interest. Even academic journals now frequently have conflict of interest rules for investigators who wish to submit articles for publication. The burden is on clinical investigators to inform themselves as early as possible in the granting or publishing process so that they can comply with the pertinent policy.

The reader may also want to be familiar with the new guideline on commercially sponsored continuing medical education. All providers of continuing medical education must be accredited by the Accreditation Council for Continuing Medical Education, which specifies certain rules that must be followed. The American Medical Association and other professional associations have also developed guidelines. Most of the rules relate to the necessity of making presentations independently of influence by the commercial sponsor. "In other words, these presentations must have an educational objective and not a marketing objective" (10). Although commercial firms may still make financial gifts, the gift must be directed to the institutional sponsor of the continuing education program to lower the overall costs of all participants and not to the individual participants. It is generally agreed that disclosure by a speaker of a relationship with the commercial sponsor is adequate to dispel the problem as long as the speaker's presentation is objective and independent from the sponsor (10).

Sanctions against clinical investigators who ignore or otherwise violate conflict of interest rules vary widely among employers. Many policies state that disciplinary action may be taken, as is done in any violation of university rules and regulations (9). Others, such as Texas (11) and California (3), provide for civil and criminal liability in certain situations. Regardless of the gravity of the violation, the astute clinical investigator will be wise to avoid even the appearance of a conflict.

RECOMMENDATIONS TO INVESTIGATORS

It is mandatory for any clinical investigator to know the policies of his or her employer, whether university, public or private hospital, or government agency. If the institution is state supported, one should also inquire as to whether there is a pertinent state statute. Policies of the professional associations with whom the investigator is affiliated should also be collected. With the relevant policies, laws, and guidelines in hand, the investigator must read and study so that these edicts are comprehended. Then, when a situation arises in which there might be a conflict of interest or the appearance of a conflict of interest, the investigator must immediately seek out his or her supervisor or the person listed in the policy as being responsible for this area. Full disclosure to the employer is the best avenue at this point. Then one must decide, in conjunction with the employer, the best method of handling the matter. No action may be needed after disclosure, although returning of compensation or equity may prove necessary. Remedies are generally not limited, and often creative problem solvers can help find solutions that will be viewed as positive and not negative to the parties involved.

REFERENCES

1. American Federation for Clinical Research (1990): Guidelines for avoiding conflict of interest. *Clin. Res.* 38:239.
2. Association of Academic Health Centers (1990): *Conflicts of Interest in Academic Health Centers.*
3. CAL. ANN. GOV'T CODE §81000-91014 (1989).
4. Chren, M., Landefeld, C., and Murray, T. (1989): Doctors, drug companies, and gifts. *JAMA* 262:3448.
5. Cornell University (n.d.): *Faculty Handbook,* p. 118.
6. Editorial (1990): Guidelines for dealing with faculty conflicts of commitment and conflicts of interest in research. *Acad. Med.* 65:487.
7. Friedman, P.J. (1991): Controlling conflict of interest. *Issues Sci. Technol.* 8:30–32.
8. Giamatti, B. (1982): The university, industry and cooperative research. *Science* 218:1278–1280.
9. Harvard University Faculty of Medicine. Policy on conflicts of interest and commitment, 1990.
10. Race, G. (1992): The winds of change in continuing medical education. *BUMC Proc.* 5:7–13.
11. TEX. REV. CIV. STAT. ANN. ART. 6252-9b (Supp. 1991).

3

Grantsmanship

Perrie M. Adams

*Office of Associate Dean for Research, University of Texas
Southwestern Medical Center at Dallas, Dallas, Texas 75235-9007*

The objectives of this chapter are to provide (a) information about sources of research funding for the clinical investigator and (b) advice regarding the preparation of the grant application itself. To meet these objectives, I discuss information regarding the funding operation of federal and private agencies. I then cover in detail the preparation of a grant proposal for application to either federal or private agencies, including format, budget, and regulatory issues.

FUNDING SOURCES

There are three basic types of funding sources underwriting the costs of clinical research. They are federal grants, private nonprofit agencies or foundations, and corporations (1). Each of these sources operates somewhat differently and requires a different approach.

Federal Grants

The federal government is the largest single source of funding for research and development. When we speak of grants, we are usually referring to grants from federal sources. Several agencies provide funding in the health area. Most of these programs fall under the Department of Health and Human Services (HHS).

There are four major agencies within HHS which have significant clinical research grant funding activities: the National Institutes of Health; the Alcohol, Drug Abuse, and Mental Health Administration (ADAMHA); the Food and Drug Administration (FDA); and the Centers for Disease Control (CDC).

The National Institutes of Health

The mandate of the NIH is to improve the health of the nation by increasing knowledge of health and disease through the conduct and support of research and research training. The majority of the NIH budget is for extramural research through grants and contracts. Approximately one-half of the grants go to medical schools; NIH is by far the most important funding agency for academic medical research.

The National Institutes of Health are divided into bureaus, institutes, and research service and support divisions. The National Library of Medicine is both a library and a research agency focusing on biomedical communications and information transfer technology. The major components of the NIH include the National Cancer Institute; the National Heart, Lung and Blood Institute; the National Institute of Arthritis and Musculoskeletal and Skin Diseases; the National Institute on Aging; the National Institute of Allergy and Infectious Diseases; the National Eye Institute; the National Institute of General Medical Sciences; the National Institute of Child Health and Human Development; the National Institute of Neurological Disorders and Stroke; the National Institute on Deafness and Other Communication Disorders; the National Institute of Diabetes and Digestive and Kidney Diseases; the National Institute of Environmental Health Sciences; the National Center for Human Genome Research; the National Institute of Dental Research; the National Center for Nursing Research; National Institute on Drug Abuse; National Institute of Mental Health; National Institute on Alcohol Abuse and Alcoholism; and the National Library of Medicine.

The National Institutes accept unsolicited proposals three times a year for their regular review cycle. Each bureau and institute publishes its grants programs in the Catalogue of Domestic Assistance. Major NIH programs do not change significantly from year to year. However, special emphases on areas of research are announced periodically. Such programs can be for either grants or contracts. Announcements for grants are called *requests for applications* (RFA) and announcements for contracts are called *requests for proposals* (RFP), and these may be found in the *NIH Guide to Grants and Contracts.*

The Alcohol, Drug Abuse, and Mental Health Administration

The Alcohol, Drug Abuse, and Mental Health Administration supports programs to deal with sociomedical problems of alcohol and drug abuse and to promote and sustain mental health and prevent mental illness. About one-half of its funds are allocated to general mental health programs and about one-third to drug abuse and alcoholism. Some of the funds are allocated through block grants to states.

The Food and Drug Administration

The Food and Drug Administration's research program is divided into four main areas: microbiology and immunology; analytical chemistry; pharmacology and pharmacokinetics; and toxicology. The FDA conducts research in its own laboratories and also supports a significant number of extramural research projects at colleges and universities, including medical schools. The FDA also sponsors research on orphan drugs (drugs that provide therapeutic benefit to a limited disease population). There are also funds available through the FDA for postmarketing studies of approved drugs.

The Centers for Disease Control

The Centers for Disease Control in Atlanta, Georgia, administer national programs for the prevention and control of communicable and vector-borne diseases and other preventable conditions. The CDC does a great deal of intramural research but does from time to time issue RFPs and RFAs for extramural research.

Foundations

After the federal government, foundations are the next largest source of research and development funds. Foundations come in all sizes and have a variety of missions or priorities. There are a few big-name foundations that we all have heard of, such as the Carnegie, the Rockefeller, the Ford, the Kaiser, the Sloane, and the Robert Wood Johnson. In fact, these foundations provided over half of all grants that were made by foundations. Yet there are many foundations of which one has never heard that may be potential sources of funding. There are several categories of foundations.

Large National Foundations

The large national foundations usually are fairly broad in scope and make fairly sizable awards. These foundations comprise the big names listed above. They are well publicized, and it is fairly easy to get information about their programs and guidelines.

Special Purpose Foundations

Special purpose foundations are those that limit their funding activities to a special category of programs. The Robert Wood Johnson Foundation and the Howard Hughes Medical Institute are examples of large, special purpose foundations limiting their programs to the health care or biomedical research area.

Regional Foundations

Regional foundations restrict their giving to a specific geographic area of the country. They may operate within only one or in more than one state.

Local Foundations

Local foundations serve the needs of a specific community or limited local area. Many local foundations bear the name of the locality, such as the Chicago Community Trust or the Cleveland Foundation. The local foundation supports a variety of worthwhile activities within the community that it serves. Many of these foundations have fairly broad guidelines for what they will fund as long as it is within their community.

Family Funds

There are a great many family foundations. The family foundation is usually fairly small and funds programs in a limited area according to the interests of the particular family.

Voluntary Health Organizations

Another source of funding is the various health organizations, such as the American Cancer Society and the American Heart Association, some of which may be set up as foundations. Although the amount of funding is not as large as from the NIH, these organizations do have a range of programs to support both research and training. Funding is usually made in the form of a grant.

Corporations

The last major source of grants and contracts is corporations. Many corporations give grants to organizations for specific activities. They also enter into contractual arrangements for research and development activities with universities and other academic agencies. Typical sponsorship is in the form of a clinical trial that is performed for a particular pharmaceutical company. Corporations are much more comfortable with contracts than they are with grants, and they are more interested in funding research that is closely related to the business priorities of the corporation. Not all corporate grants are in the form of money. Equipment donations are becoming more common. In fact, there have been some modifications of the tax laws to encourage corporations to give equipment to support research at institutions of higher education.

GRANT PREPARATION

The writing of a grant application requires the same care and skill that are involved in preparing a manuscript for publication (2). The major difference is in the format required by the sponsor and the level of detail in specific sections of the application. The major sections of a proposal are shown in Table 1.

Specific Aims

The first section usually is called the Specific Aims. This section should include a clearly stated outline of the proposed studies. The aims of the proposed research should be a logical presentation of feasible experiments related to the hypothesis being tested. Depending on the scope of the project, the number of aims should be limited to three to five.

Background and Significance

The background section should include a review of the relevant literature related to the problem area under study. The review should be a critical one in which gaps are identified and the relevance to the proposed aims is clearly addressed. This section does not have to include an exhaustive review of the literature but rather should focus on the most important articles related to the proposed aims of the grant and the hypotheses being tested.

TABLE 1. *Major sections of a grant proposal for clinical research*

- Specific aims
- Background and significance
- Preliminary data
- Experimental design
- Methods and procedures
- Statistical analysis
- Human subject involvement
- Budget

Preliminary Data

The inclusion of preliminary data with the grant application is considered by most to be essential for funding success. The extent of this section will vary depending upon the nature of the application and the seniority of the applicant. Young investigators applying for new investigator type grants are generally not expected to have had the opportunity to do extensive research on the topic, and therefore fewer preliminary data are needed. In contrast, the more established scientist will need to demonstrate that the proposed work has merit based on the experiments already conducted.

In any case, it is important for the preliminary data section to demonstrate the feasibility of the proposed experiments. In the case of the young investigator, or where an investigator is moving into an area in which the scientist is not well identified, the preliminary data can provide evidence of the applicant's ability to perform the technical aspects of the proposed studies. Tables and graphs to illustrate the findings to date are very useful.

Finally, the results of the preliminary experiments should be related to the proposed studies and thus provide an additional opportunity to identify the significance of the proposed work.

Experimental Design

The description of the experimental design of the proposed studies is a critical section of the proposal. It is also the section that frequently receives the least attention from the applicant.

In this section a logical presentation of the proposed experiments should be given. From the presentation the reader should have a clear picture of the rationale for the studies and how each relates to the hypotheses being tested. The design of each experiment should identify the treatment conditions, the number of subjects, and the independent and dependent variables.

One should avoid proposing parallel experiments running concurrently because this tends to make the reader think that the project may be unfocused. It is much better to propose a series of experiments, each of which builds on the results of the prior one. This allows the reader to follow the applicant's logic and relate the studies to the specific aims. It is also important to relate the experimental design to the statistical analysis section of the grant to demonstrate to the reviewer that the writer has given careful thought to how the data will be analyzed.

Methods and Procedures

The methods section is the part of the grant where the investigator gives the details of how the the experiments will be carried out. Most granting agencies such as the NIH have restricted the number of pages allowed for the methods section. Regardless of the limits, keep this section reasonably short. Avoid giving too much detail unless you are discussing a new technology or methods not previously published.

One of the major goals of the methods section is to provide clear evidence that the proposed techniques can be performed. If the reviewer doubts the investigator's ability to perform the methods required to carry out the experiments, funding is unlikely.

It is also critical to avoid techniques with inherent limitations that could make the next experimental step impossible. This amounts to building the proposal on a "house of cards" so that, if one aspect were to fall, the whole proposal would collapse.

Last, present a timetable or flow diagram of the experiments to give the reviewer a visual picture of how the studies relate to each other and the time course for the project period requested.

Statistical Analysis

As noted previously under "Experimental Design," it is important to relate the design of the experiments to how the data will be analyzed. Too frequently the applicant describes in detail the methods but fails to discuss how the data will be analyzed.

The applicant is strongly advised to consult with a statistician when planning the experimental design to ensure that the appropriate statistical methods will be used. This advance planning will reduce the likelihood that data are collected in a manner that makes subsequent analysis difficult.

In discussing the statistical analysis, clearly identify the dependent and independent variables to be analyzed. Based upon the nature of these data, you should select the appropriate type of analysis to be used.

In describing the data, include a measure of variability, usually the standard deviation, along with the measure of central tendency (e.g., mean). Present the data in the same manner as used in the statistical analysis and provide graphs or tables to illustrate and visually summarize the findings.

Human Subject Involvement

In this chapter, the topic of human subject involvement as it relates to the grant application is briefly discussed. A more detailed discussion of human subject issues appears in Chapter 4.

The application should describe in some detail how the human subject will be involved in the proposed studies. In describing the participation of the human subject, the investigator should be certain to address the extent to which male and female subjects will be included. If one gender is excluded, state the justification on which the decision was based. The rationale for exclusion should be based on science, not convenience or availability. Similarly, the exclusion of a minority group should be avoided unless there is clear justification. A detailed protocol that describes what the human subject is asked to do should be included. Include those procedures that are being done for the research protocol and exclude those that are part of clinical management.

In the protocol the sources of research material (e.g., tissue, blood) should be clearly described. The risks related to the acquisition of these materials should also be clearly stated.

If there are other risks associated with human subject participation, they should be described in both the protocol and the consent form. A discussion of the benefits and the relationship of the benefits to the risks of participation should be included. Last, a description of the recruitment methods to be used and the process of obtaining informed consent should be included for each experiment in the application. Some funding agencies require a copy of the consent document to be used, whereas others require only the approval date of the institutional review board.

Budget

The most important point to make in the presentation of the budget is the justification. Each aspect of the budget (i.e., personnel, equipment, supplies) must be fully justified. Be specific about the role of each individual named under the personnel section. Try to avoid "to be named" salary positions. Such positions are too easy for the reviewers to eliminate. The emphasis should be on personnel needed to conduct the science not on support staff.

Be very explicit regarding the equipment and supplies requested. Provide accurate costs and strong justification, especially for equipment items. Minimize the amount requested for travel, and state the specific needs for the travel funds.

Renovation costs are generally seen as an institutional responsibility and therefore are generally not supported through grant funds. Check with the Office of Grants Management or the sponsored programs office to obtain the appropriate indirect cost rate and the current fringe benefit rate.

It is important to inquire into possible institutional rate changes or per diem rate changes that may be going into effect in the future; these will affect the budgets of later years. Similarly, factor into the future-year budgets an inflationary effect on the different categories (salaries and supplies in particular). It is important that the budget in future years of the project fit the proposed work so that the reviewer has a clear picture of not only what is planned but what it will cost.

Summary

In closing, the following suggestions are given as grantsmanship "DOs."

1. Have others read the proposal in draft form and provide critical feedback.
2. Allow ample time to prepare the grant application and to obtain all institutional approvals (e.g., investigational review board, radiation safety committee).
3. Pay particular attention to the overall appearance of the grant, including type size, font selection, margins, figures, tables, and required formats.
4. Strive for clearness and brevity throughout the application.
5. Verify all your references for completeness and accuracy.

In a similar fashion, the following "DON'Ts" are given as closing advice to the grant writer.

1. Do not exceed the page limitations or ignore the format specifications set by the sponsoring agencies.
2. Do not abuse the use of appendix materials.
3. Do not propose too ambitious a set of studies relative to the time frame and budget of the proposal.
4. Do not cite too many abstracts in the application, particularly if critical to the hypothesis, since many never get published.
5. Do not assume that the reader will know all the relevant literature in the specified area of research.

REFERENCES

1. Hinds, J. and Battles, J. (1988): *Development of Grant and Contract Proposals.* University of Texas Southwestern Medical Center, Office of Grants Management.
2. Sontheimer, R.D. and Bergstresser, P.R. (1991): The ABCs of research grant writing: the advice of two grant reviewers. *J Invest Dermatol* 97(2):165–168.

4

Protection of Human Subjects and Protocol Preparation

Perrie M. Adams

*Office of Associate Dean for Research, University of Texas
Southwestern Medical Center at Dallas, Dallas, Texas 75235-9007*

The performance of clinical research is focused on the participation of human subjects, whether they be patients or healthy volunteers. It is essential for the clinical investigator to be aware of the importance of ensuring that the rights and welfare of these human subjects be adequately protected.

This chapter provides the clinical researcher with the basic ethical principles behind the regulations developed to ensure the protection of human subjects in research. I discuss the elements of a consent form, the factors essential to informed consent, and the protections needed for such special populations of human subjects as children or pregnant women. Finally, I discuss the integration of human research issues with the grant proposal and the protocol itself.

BACKGROUND

From the time of Hippocrates physicians have been charged with protecting their patients from harm. The ethical principles that have guided the conduct of clinical investigation have revolved about (a) respect for persons, (b) beneficence, and (c) justice.

These principles form the basis for the regulations that today determine how the rights of human subjects in research are protected. The foundation for these regulations was the language adopted by the World Medical Assembly held in 1964 in Helsinki, Finland. The discussions at the Helsinki meeting resulted in the publication of the following guidelines for physicians conducting human research (4).

1. Biomedical research on human subjects must be done in a manner that conforms with acceptable scientific principles. Further, this research should be founded upon adequate preclinical research on animals and on a thorough review of the scientific literature.

2. Each experimental procedure to be conducted involving a human subject should be described in a protocol that must be reviewed by an independent committee.

3. Only qualified scientists should conduct human investigation, and the responsibility for the human subject should always rest with a medically qualified individual, not the subject, regardless of the subject's having given consent.

4. The importance of the research must be in proportion to the risks to the human subjects participating.

5. The predictable risks in a project must be assessed relative to the foreseeable benefits to the subject or to society. Concern for the welfare of the subject takes precedence over the interest of science or society.

6. Rights of the personal integrity of the subject must be respected. This includes the right to privacy as well as physical and psychological well-being.

7. In obtaining informed consent, particular attention should be paid to the avoidance of possible dependency relationships involving the subject and investigator.

8. In the case of incompetence, whether mental or physical, where informed consent is not possible, a legal guardian should be asked to provide the informed consent.

9. The research protocol should state the ethical considerations involved in the research, and these principles must be complied with by the investigators.

RESPECT FOR PERSONS

The principle of respect for persons is based upon the ethical premise that the individual has certain rights to autonomy. In addition, the principle includes the premise that an individual with diminished autonomy should be given additional protection. The right of autonomy or self-determination translates into the requirement of asking permission of an individual before anyone can touch or do anything to the individual. In the case of human research, the principle of respect for persons becomes the basis for the practice of obtaining informed consent.

BENEFICENCE

The principle of beneficence includes the Hippocratic Oath mandate of "Do no harm" and the maximizing of benefits while minimizing risks. Physicians pledge to act for the benefit of patients. Similarly, by accepting public funds for research efforts, the clinical investigator has an obligation to promote good by contributing new knowledge. Therefore, the investigator has a dual obligation based on the principle of beneficence: To do no harm to the subject and to contribute new information to society.

JUSTICE

The principle of justice requires that we treat individuals fairly and that each person is given what is due or owed (1). In the context of protecting human subjects, the concept of justice is used in the form of distributive justice. Distributive justice is concerned with the distribution of scarce benefits where there is some competition for these benefits (2). Distributive justice also relates to the distribution of burden, particularly as it becomes necessary to impose burdens on a few rather than all members of a seemingly similar class of persons. This principle requires a fair sharing of risks and benefits. It is of particular importance in the issue of the selection of research participants.

BASIC DEFINITIONS

Before we go further it is important to establish some definitions essential in a discussion of human research. The definitions were developed as part of the regulations set forth by the Department of Health and Human Services (3).

A *human subject* is defined as "a living individual about whom an investigator conducting research obtains (a) data through intervention or interaction with the individual, or (b) identifiable private information." Intervention might include a physical procedure such as a venipuncture or a drug treatment or a manipulation of the subject's environment. Interaction might include direct interpersonal contact or communication with the subject. Private information would include that information about the subject that would normally be expected not to occur or to be recorded. It would also include information about the subject that would normally be expected to be held confidential (e.g., the medical record).

Research is defined as "a systematic investigation designed to develop or contribute to generalized knowledge." This definition holds whether the research is funded or not.

Minimal risk means that "the risks of harm anticipated in the proposed research are not greater, considering probability and magnitude, than those ordinarily encountered in daily life or during the performance of routine physical or psychological examinations or tests."

Given these definitions, it is the function of the Institutional Review Board (IRB) to oversee the protection of human subjects in research as defined above. The IRB is mandated by federal regulations to perform this oversight function (3). It is the function of the IRB to assure that (a) risks to human subjects are minimized and reasonable in relation to anticipated benefits, (b) there is informed consent, and (c) the rights and welfare of subjects are maintained in other ways as well.

THE CRITERIA FOR IRB APPROVAL

To obtain IRB approval for a protocol involving human subjects, it must meet the following criteria.

1.   The risks to the subjects are minimized by (a) using procedures consistent with sound research design and (b) not exposing the subject to unnecessary risks.

2.   The risks are reasonable in relation to benefits.

3.   The selection of the subjects is equitable.

4.   Informed consent is obtained.

5.   Consent documentation is acceptable.

6.   Data are monitored.

7.   Privacy and confidentiality are respected and protected.

Protocols are reviewed for each of these criteria. Recommended changes in the consent form and protocol are provided to the investigator. After further review, if the contingencies are met, final approval is given.

For the subject participating in clinical research, the consent form is the primary source of information regarding the study. This document states in understandable language what the study is about and what participation involves.

The general requirements of informed consent include the following:

1. No investigator may use a human subject in a study without a legally effective informed consent.

2. The prospective subject must have the opportunity to consider whether to participate or not under conditions that minimize coercion or undue influence.

3. Information must be given to the subject in understandable language.

4. There must be no exculpatory language that requires the subject to waive or seem to waive his or her rights.

The basic elements of the consent form given the subject should include (a) a clear statement that this is a research study (including purpose, duration, and procedures that are experimental); (b) a description of foreseeable risks; (c) a description of the benefits; (d) a description of alternatives to the procedures; (e) a description of how confidentiality will be protected; (f) an explanation of compensation/treatment for injury, should it occur; (g) identification of whom to contact with questions related to the research, the subject's rights, and injury or adverse reactions; and (h) an explanation of the right to refuse and withdraw from the study.

In addition to the above basic elements of a consent form, there are others that should be considered depending upon the nature of the study. These additional elements include (a) possible unforeseeable risks, (b) the circumstances under which the investigator might terminate the subject's participation, (c) additional costs to the subject, (d) the consequences of a subject's withdrawing from the study, (e) information that the results of new findings will be provided, and (f) the number of subjects in the study.

The IRB may require some or all of these elements for a particular protocol. There may be circumstances in which the IRB would waive informed consent completely. To waive consent, the IRB must conclude and document that the research (a) is to be conducted by or is subject to approval of a state or local government and is designed to study aspects of the Social Security Act programs and (b) could not be practicably carried out without the waiver.

An IRB may also determine that elements of the consent process or the obtaining of informed consent may be waived provided that:

1. The research involves no more than minimal risk,

2. Waiver of consent will not adversely affect the subject's rights,

3. The research could not practicably be performed without the waiver.

4. When appropriate, the subject will be provided pertinent information about the study afterward.

Except in the above circumstances written informed consent would be required. The consent form should be signed by the subject, the person obtaining consent, and a witness. A legally authorized person could sign for the subject, if appropriate.

On occasion the IRB may waive the actual signing of a consent form if it determines that (a) the only record linking the subject to the research is the written consent form and the principal risk is loss of confidentiality or (b) the research risk is minimal and involves no procedures for which written consent is normally obtained outside the research context.

EXEMPT RESEARCH AREAS

Certain types of research are identified in the federal regulations as qualifying for exemption.

1. Research conducted in educational settings involving normal educational practices including (a) research on educational instruction strategies or (b) the effectiveness of instructional techniques, curricula, or classroom management methods.

2. Research involving the use of educational tests if the information is recorded in a manner that cannot be directly linked to the subject.

3. Research involving survey or questionnaire procedures except when (a) identifiers are linked to the subject, (b) there is potential risk of criminal or civil liability if responses were made known, or (c) the research involves sensitive aspects of the subject's own behavior.

4. Research involving the collection or study of existing data, documents, specimens, or records.

TABLE 1. *Criteria for expedited review*

- No more than minimal risk
- Research procedures
  —Specimens from hair, nails, and teeth
  —Urine or stool samples
  —Noninvasive routine tests on adults
  —Blood samples by venipuncture in adults
  —Plaque and calculus samples
  —Voice recordings
  —Exercise
  —Behavior or characteristics measures
  —Existing data, records, or specimens
  —Drugs, devices if IND or IDE is not required

EXPEDITED REVIEW RESEARCH

The federal regulations of 1983 established an expedited review procedure to facilitate the IRB review and approval of selected types of research. To qualify for this type of review the research must be restricted to minimal risk and fall within a list of specific procedures. The IRB has authority to review some or all of the research that falls under the listed procedures if the overall risk is no more than minimal. Expedited review can also be used to assess minor changes in a protocol that has already received IRB approval. The procedures currently identified as eligible for expedited review are given in Table 1.

SPECIAL POPULATION PROTECTIONS

Fetuses, Pregnant Women, and *In Vitro* Fertilization

Federal regulations provide additional safeguards for the protection of this population through the establishment of special advisory boards within the federal government. In addition, IRBs are responsible for assuring that no research on fetuses or pregnant women or with *in vitro* fertilization is conducted unless preclinical research on animals and studies with nonpregnant subjects have been completed. Further, the following considerations must be met.

1. The research activity will be conducted for the purpose of meeting the health needs of the pregnant woman or the fetus, the risks to the fetus will be minimal, and the least possible risk will be present.

2. Individuals involved in the research will have no part in (a) decisions related to the timing, method, or termination procedures of the pregnancy and (b) determination of the viability of the fetus at termination of the pregnancy.

3. No change in procedure that may cause greater than minimal risk either to the pregnant woman or to the fetus will be made in the methods used for terminating the pregnancy solely for the research activity.

4. No offer of monetary or other inducement will be allowed in an effort to terminate the pregnancy for the purposes of the research activity.

5. Research with pregnant subjects must include legally competent participation by both the mother and father with informed consent regarding the possible effect on the fetus. The father's consent is not required if (a) the research is directed at the health needs of the mother, (b) his identity or whereabouts is unknown, (c) he is not reasonably available, or (d) the pregnancy is the result of rape.

6. Research that involves the fetus *in utero* may not occur unless (a) the research is designed to help the direct health needs of the fetus and the risk is minimal, (b) the risk to the fetus is minimal and the knowledge to be gained could not be obtained by other means, and (c) the mother and father are competent and give legally informed consent.

The father's consent may be waived if the conditions described above (5a–d) are met. Similar protections are in order for the fetus *ex utero* and include nonviable fetuses. These protections stress the importance of respect for the fetus as an individual and the contribution to biomedical knowledge that could be obtained only through the proposed research.

Protection for Prisoners

Because of the inherently constraining environment inhabited by prisoners, additional protections were provided to protect them from possible coercion or undue influence with respect to their participation in research. The composition of an IRB and its relationship to the prison are important considerations. A majority of the IRB membership must have no association with the prison. Further, at least one IRB member must be a prisoner or a prisoner representative.

The IRB must determine that the following conditions are met.

1. Any possible advantages to the prisoner as a result of participation in the research are not so great as to influence the prisoner's judgment of the risks of the research.

2. The risks of participating in the research are commensurate with the level of risk that a nonprisoner would accept.

3. Selection procedures are fair and equitable for all prisoners and not subject to arbitrary intervention by prison staff or other prisoners.

4. The information regarding the research is presented in a manner understandable to the subjects.

5. Adequate assurance is made to prevent parole boards from using information related to the prisoner's participation in research for making parole decisions.

6. The IRB will inform the prisoner participating in research of the need for follow-up study or care and that provisions for providing the care or follow-up have been made.

In addition to the above provisions the IRB must consider the type of research proposed and whether it qualifies for the inclusion of prisoners. The specific types of research considered appropriate for prisoner participation include, first, studies of the cause, effect, and process of incarceration and of criminal behavior. These studies must carry no more than minimal risk and must be no more than inconvenient for the subjects. Second, prisoners might participate in studies on conditions that affect them as a class. These would include clinical trials on vaccines and other studies on hepatitis, as well as research on such psychological disorders as alcoholism, drug abuse, and violent behavior. Third, they may engage in research that has the intent and reasonable probability of improving the health or well-being of the prisoner.

Review of these studies generally will require special review by experts in penology and approval by the Secretary of Health and Human Services.

Protection for Children

Because of the inability of the child to give informed consent, added protections have been incorporated into the regulations for human research. These added safeguards allow the following.

1. Research in children not involving greater than minimal risk can occur if the child assents and the parents or guardian gives permission.

2. Research involving more than minimal risk but having the prospect of direct benefit to the individual subject can occur if (a) the risk is justified by the likely benefit to the child, (b) the anticipated benefit-to-risk ratio is as favorable as the alternatives to the child, and (c) the assent of the child and the permission of the parents are solicited.

3. Research that involves greater than minimal risk and no likelihood of direct benefit to the child but possible generalizable new knowledge can occur if the risk is a minor increase over minimal risk, the intervention presents risks that are commensurate with the experiences the child is expected to have given the medical condition, the intervention is likely to provide generalizable knowledge that will be of importance to the understanding of the subject's disease or condition, and the assent of the child and permission of the parents are solicited.

PROTOCOL PREPARATION

In addition to the consent form for a clinical study, a detailed protocol is needed for the IRB to review. The protocol should include the following.

1. *Purpose*—A statement of the study objectives.

2. *Background*—A brief review of the state of development of the drug, device, or concepts to be studied.

3. *Concise summary of the project*—A brief description of the proposed study written at a layman's language level.

4. *Criteria for the inclusion of subjects*—A description of the characteristics of the subject population and the inclusion criteria and an explanation of the rationale for the use of special classes of subjects who are considered vulnerable.

5. *Criteria for the exclusion of subjects*—A description of the characteristics that would exclude a person from study inclusion.

6. *Sources of research material*—Identification of the sources of the research material obtained from individuals in the form of specimens, records, or data and an indication of whether the material or data will be obtained specifically for research purposes or whether existing specimens, records, or data will be used.

7. *Recruitment of subjects*—A description of the plans for the recruitment of subjects and the consent procedures and identification of who will obtain the informed consent, the nature of the information to be provided, and how it will be documented.

8. *Potential risks*—A description of any potential risks or discomforts for the subjects and an assessment of their likelihood and seriousness.

9. *Special precautions*—A description of the procedures for protecting against any potential risks and an assessment of their likely effectiveness. Where appropriate, provisions for ensuring necessary medical intervention in the event of adverse effects to the subjects are discussed.

10. *Procedures to maintain confidentiality*—A discussion of how the confidentiality of the participating subjects will be maintained. Information on where copies of the consent forms will be maintained and under what circumstances information about an individual research subject would be disclosed is included.

11. *Potential benefits*—A description of and assessment of the potential benefits of the study; specifically, discussion of the benefits relative to the human subjects involved, other individuals having similar problems, and society in general.

12. *Risk/benefit assessment*—A discussion of why the risks to subjects are reasonable in relation to the benefits anticipated from the study. The

greater the personal risk of the research, the greater the need to demonstrate the opportunity for direct benefits to the subject.

THE INTEGRATION OF HUMAN RESEARCH ISSUES WITH THE GRANT PROPOSAL

The format of a grant application will dictate where within the application the issues related to human subjects will be located. The methodology section may provide the most appropriate location for the description of the protocol. Issues related to subject recruitment and informed consent are best addressed in a separate section of the application which highlights these issues. A copy of the consent form approved by the IRB, although not usually required, could be included as an appendix item.

CONCLUSION

As important as clinical investigation is for the progress of medical science and patient care, it is critical that the human research subject be given every protection from harm. This chapter was written with the goal of providing the essential information necessary to protect the human subjects participating in research protocols. Providing these protections to the subjects and obtaining their informed consent does not jeopardize the study but in fact can lead to better research.

REFERENCES

1. Beauchamp, T.L. (1978): Distributive justice and morally relevant differences. In: *The National Commission for the Protection of Human Subjects of Biomedical and Behavioral Research: The Belmont Report: Ethical Prinicipals and Guidelines for the Protection of Human Subjects of Research.Washington*, DC. DHEW Publication 78-0013.
2. Levine, R.J. (1986):*Ethics and Regulation of Clinical Research.* Urban and Schwarzenberg, Baltimore, MD.
3. U.S. Department of Health and Human Services (1983): *Department. of Health and Human Services Rules and Regulations.*45CFR46. U.S. Government Printing Office, Washington, DC.
4. World Medical Assembly (1975): *World Medical Association Declaration of Helsinki: Recommendations Guiding Medical Doctors in Biomedical Research Involving Human Subjects.* Helsinki, Finland, 1964, Tokyo, Japan.

5

Designing Clinical Research

Robert W. Haley

Division of Epidemiology, Department of Internal Medicine, University of Texas Southwestern Medical Center at Dallas, Dallas, Texas 75235-8874

Conducting successful clinical research projects requires careful planning before the collection of data begins. Although the planning process comes naturally to some new investigators, others must learn how to plan research by observing their mentors and reading books on research design. The purpose of this chapter is to provide an overview of the design process to accelerate the learning curve and make new investigators productive in a shorter time.

Designing and carrying out a clinical research project can be divided into 16 discrete steps (Tables 1 and 2). The first 10 are the steps required in planning the study before data collection begins (Table 1). The final 6 are the execution steps carried out in the data collection, analysis, and publishing phase (Table 2). Ideally, the investigator should be aware of and address all of these steps in the design phase to ensure the feasibility and success of the project. This chapter will deal with each of the 16 steps in turn.

TABLE 1. *Steps 1-10 in designing and carrying out a clinical research project: The planning steps*

1. Develop good ideas for research.
2. Write the objectives and establish priorities.
3. Define the variables needed.
4. Define the study population.
5. Refine the objectives into written, testable hypotheses.
6. Anticipate error and bias.
7. Develop the study design.
8. Estimate the sample size needed.
9. Write a research protocol for review.
10. Plan the data collection process.

STEP 1: DEVELOP GOOD IDEAS FOR RESEARCH

The single most important step in successful clinical research is to come up with an important idea to study. A research career is simply too short to spend time researching unimportant questions. Moreover, answering important questions leads to funded grants, scientific publications, and professional advancement.

Formulating important questions requires experience in the clinical field to be studied and interaction with other experienced investigators. From one's own experience or with the help of other investigators, the new investigator must ask, "What is an important question that, if I could answer it, would greatly advance the understanding or practice in my field?" The seminal questions in any field tend to change as research advances. They can best be identified by such approaches as attending national research meetings, seeking insights from experienced colleagues, and simply working in a field for a number of years.

A frequent mistake of new investigators is to start from the wrong end of the research process in formulating research questions. For instance, one should not

TABLE 2. *Steps 11-16 in designing and carrying out a clinical research project: The execution steps*

11. Manage and monitor data collection.
12. Manage the database.
13. Analyze the results into tables and graphs.
14. Test the hypothesis with correct statistical tests.
15. Generate additional tables and graphs to explain the findings.
16. Publish the results in a scientific journal.

adopt a research method or technique and ask, "What interesting measurements can I make with this powerful laboratory technique?" Similarly, one should not obtain an existing clinical database with the idea, "I'll bet I can analyze this database and answer some interesting questions." Efforts that begin with methods or databases and proceed to questions rarely generate important conclusions. Instead, one should determine the important questions in the field and design the methods and databases needed to answer them.

Once an exciting idea has been identified, the new investigators should review the scientific literature and discuss the idea with mentors and colleagues. These days, a complete scientific literature review can be conducted rapidly through use of the National Library of Medicine's MEDLINE database, which can be accessed by computer in any medical library and via personal computer and modem from home. After reading the titles and abstracts of articles indexed under appropriate key words, the researcher should go to the library and read the articles considered most relevant to the research. This will determine whether others have attempted to address the subject, identify research approaches and methods used successfully or unsuccessfully by prior investigators, and provide additional contextual information of importance in designing the project. Armed with knowledge from the literature, one is then in the position to discuss the subject meaningfully with others. The discussion process helps the investigator refine the idea and think through complex issues or impediments to the research.

Once the idea has been thoroughly researched and discussed, it is often necessary to limit its scope before beginning the project. Often what seemed like a simple idea at first mushrooms into a grandiose plan that is not feasible. The researcher must realistically assess the idea and narrow its scope to something that can be accomplished with the time and resources that might realistically be obtained.

STEP 2: WRITE THE OBJECTIVES AND ESTABLISH PRIORITIES

Early in the planning process, the researcher must make a list of all of the objectives that are to be accomplished. When the objectives are not formally written, often there is an unrecognized confusion over how many objectives there are and exactly what they are. Only by writing them down in formally worded statements can they be clarified. The new investigator is usually surprised to find, when writing down the objective of the study, that there were really two or three somewhat different objectives being interchangeably discussed when the original research idea was being formulated.

Once all of the objectives are identified, they must be rewritten in order of priority and relative importance. In some instances, the competition among objectives is so extreme that two or more objectives can simply not be addressed in the same study. This will become crucial to the design in later steps because, almost always, the several objectives will compete with each other for study resources, such as sample size, financial resources, and personnel time. It is therefore important to set the priorities among objectives before going further in the design.

STEP 3: DEFINE THE VARIABLES NEEDED

Once the objectives are formally written, the investigator develops a plan for accomplishing the objectives, that is, for answering the questions entailed by the objectives. Generally, the first decision in developing the plan is to enumerate the variables that will have to be measured to answer the questions. After enumerating all of the variables, later steps will deal with defining the variables more fully, anticipating problems in measuring and comparing the variables, and formulating a study design in which the measurements can be used for drawing causal inferences.

In all studies, variables may serve any of three different uses (Table 3). They may serve as dependent variables, independent variables, or extraneous variables.

The **dependent variables** are the measures of the outcomes of the study. They are often referred to as outcome variables, response variables, disease variables, or effect variables. They constitute the effect in the cause-and-effect relationship.

The **independent variables** are the presumed causal variables in the cause-and-effect relationship. They are often referred to in different contexts as treatment variables, causal variables, classification variables, and factor variables. In epidemiological studies they are often referred to as risk factors. In experiments, the independent variable is assigned by the investigator and is under the investigator's control, whereas in observational studies it is not.

The **extraneous variables** are additional variables not of direct interest to the investigator but that might adversely affect the study unless they are accounted for in the design or the analysis. They are often referred to as confounding variables, biasing variables, noise variables, co-variables, or effect modifiers (see Step 6 below).

TABLE 3. *The 3 strategic uses that variables may serve in a research project*

Dependent variables

> Also called: outcome variables
> response variables
> effect variables

Independent variables

> Also called: treatment variables
> classification variables
> causal variables
> risk factors

Extraneous variables

> Also called: confounding variables
> biasing variables
> noise variables
> co-variables

As an example, in a clinical trial to determine the efficacy of an investigational drug for preventing angina pectoris, the group to which the patient was assigned (drug or placebo) would be the independent variable; whether the patient subsequently experienced angina pectoris (or the number of attacks) would be the dependent variable; and such measurements as the cause of the anginal pain (coronary artery disease versus valvular heart disease), the extent and severity of coronary arterial narrowing, and the number of previous myocardial infarctions might be extraneous variables of interest.

After brainstorming and discussing with colleagues the choice of potential variables, the investigator should make a list of the variables of interest in the study. When the list has been narrowed down to the best variables for each of the three uses, the investigator should write a formal definition for each variable, including the valid codes, or values, with which the variable will be coded in the data collection process. When studying diseases, the dependent variable is often a measure of whether or not a patient developed the disease, and the definition of this variable is called the **case definition.** The wording of the variable definitions is extremely important and should be carefully formulated because these definitions will be applied literally in classifying patients in the data collection process. If the definitions are too broad or unclear, this may result in serious misclassifications that could bias the study results. Often the definitions will need to be discussed among collaborators or with a mentor to ensure that they are precisely and appropriately stated.

After they have been defined, a concise description of how each variable will be measured should also be written. For some variables, this will be a short statement, but for others it might require a several-page description of laboratory methods or equipment configurations.

In defining and describing the variables, the investigator must also anticipate the statistical analysis that will be applied at the end of the study. While many new investigators find it uncomfortable to think of analyzing the data before it is even collected, at least a broad outline of the analysis is essential before finalizing the definitions of the variables. Some investigators even go through the motions of writing out the methods and results sections of their scientific paper in mock fashion before data collection begins, imagining what they are predicting to find to ensure that the list of variables and codes is going to be adequate for their needs. Such advance scrutiny of the variables is important because the approach that can be used for the statistical analysis is determined to a large extent by the types of variables and their codes measured in the study.

There are basically four types of variables, that is, four types of scales on which variables in clinical research are usually measured (Table 4). The four types of variables corresponding to these scales are **two-categoried (dichotomous)** variables, **multicategoried, nominal** variables, **multicategoried, ordered (or ordinal)** variables, and **continuous (or interval)** variables (Table 4). In general, dichotomous categorical variables are the easiest to collect and analyze but may not give enough information for some clinical studies. Continuous variables are often more difficult to analyze but may be necessary to answer some research questions. These will be discussed in more detail under Step 14.

STEP 4: DEFINE THE STUDY POPULATION

While determining the variables to be measured, the investigator simultaneously defines the population to be studied. In clinical research, the population is generally a group of patients found in the hospital, admitted to a clinic, or simply identified in the population. In defining the population to be studied, however, it is frequently not sufficient to include simply a group of patients that can be conveniently assembled.

To guide the definition of the study population, one must ask "What is the **target universe**?" or "What is the group of people to which the study's results are to be generalized at the end of the study?" The investigator should write a description of the target universe.

TABLE 4. *The 4 main types, or forms, of variables used in clinical research*

Categorical, dichotomous

> The variable has only 2 categories, such as DIED ("yes"/"no") or SEX ("male"/"female").

Categorical, multicategoried, nominal

> The variable has more than 2 categories but they are naming (nominal) and not intrinsically ordered, such as COLOR ("white"/"black"/"green"/"red") or SERVICE ("Medicine"/"Surgery"/"Obstetrics"/"Pediatrics").

Categorical, multicategoried, ordered

> The variable has more than 2 categories and they are intrinsically ordered (ordinal), such as TITER ("non-reactive"/"1:8"/"1:16"/"1:32"/"1:64") or AGE GROUPS ("18-34"/"35-49"/"50-74"/"75 and older").

Continuous (or interval)

> The variable is measured on a continuous scale, such as TEMPERATURE (in degrees F), or has a large number of discrete, ordered values, such as AGE (in years).

Once the target universe has been described, the investigator must decide whether to enroll all members of the target universe into the study or to select a smaller sample of them. In most research, it is not feasible to study all members of the target universe, and therefore samples of the target universe are almost always studied. In selecting the sample, the investigator must weigh the alternative types of samples carefully to ensure that the final results can be generalized back to the target universe.

There are three basic kinds of samples (Table 5). A **statistical sample** is a sample of the target universe selected by some process of random numbers. Although there are a number of techniques for random sampling, the defining characteristic of a statistical sample is that all members of the target universe have an equal probability of being selected into the sample. The advantage of a statistical sample is that the results obtained in the sample will be true of the target population within a range of error that can be calculated from the information in the sample. Its disadvantage is that it is often infeasible when the target universe is ill-defined or when there are no lists or other means for selecting a random sample.

The second type of sample is a **convenience sample**. It generally comprises a group of patients from the target universe, nonrandomly selected, who could be conveniently enrolled in the study and who seem to make up a reasonably representative sample of the target universe. Since the members of a convenience sample were not selected by a true random sampling method, one will not have the same degree of assurance that the results can be generalized to the target universe as one would have with a random sample. However, many convenience samples are free enough of obvious biases to provide accurate estimates of the characteristics of their target universe. Often when using a convenience sample, it is helpful, or necessary, to perform analyses comparing characteristics of the convenience sample with those of the target universe to determine whether biases exist and, if so, their extent.

The third type of sample is referred to as a **chunk**. When random sampling is infeasible and there are no convenience samples to be had, an investigator may be forced to study a group of subjects whose similarity to the target universe is unknown and possibly unknowable. When studying a chunk, the investigator must admit that the results might give a highly misleading picture of what is true in the target universe. On the other hand, there are many circumstances in which biological characteristics or effects are so universal in the population that the degree of similarity of the sample to the target universe is of no importance. In such instances, studying a chunk of patients gives quite satisfactory results and may prove far less expensive than either a convenience sample or a random sample.

TABLE 5. *The 3 types of samples for making efficient estimates of parameters in a large target universe*

Statistical sample

Selected by a system of random numbers. The results are true of the target universe with known error.

Convenience sample

Selected by a convenient, though non-random, method. The results are probably true of the target universe but the error is not precisely known.

Chunk

Selected by a convenient, though non-random, method. There is no way to tell whether the results are true of the target universe, and the error is entirely unknown.

STEP 5: REFINE THE OBJECTIVES INTO WRITTEN, TESTABLE HYPOTHESES

Once the objectives have been written, the variables defined, and the study population determined, it is necessary to refine the written objectives into a set of written, testable hypotheses. This must be done before the study design can be determined.

Basically, an hypothesis is simply a **prediction** of how the variables will be found to be associated in the final statistical analysis. It differs from the written objective in that it is stated in terms of the actual statistical associations that will be found among the precisely defined variables formulated in Step 3.

The hypothesis may be stated in one of two forms. Statisticians generally prefer what is called the **null hypothesis**. For example, in a study to test the efficacy of a new drug in treating hypertension, the null hypothesis (abbreviated H_0:) might be stated as follows:

> H_0: The mean diastolic blood pressure in the treated group will be *no different from* that in the untreated group.

Notice that this statement of the null hypothesis is **nondirectional**, that is, the null hypothesis would be rejected (proved untrue) if the blood pressure in the treated group was found to be either higher or lower than that in the untreated group. The corresponding **alternative hypothesis** (abbreviated H_A:) would be written as follows:

> H_A: The mean diastolic blood pressure in the treated group will be *different* (either higher or lower) from that in the untreated group.

For a nondirectional hypothesis like this, a **two-tailed** statistical test must be used in the analysis.

In contrast, the null hypothesis may sometimes be expressed in a **directional** manner, as follows:

> H_0: The mean diastolic blood pressure in the treated group will be *no lower than* that in the untreated group.

The corresponding **alternative hypothesis** would be written as follows:

H_A: The mean diastolic blood pressure in the treated group will be *lower than* that in the untreated group.

For a directional hypothesis like this, a **one-tailed** statistical test must be used in the analysis.

The point of this discussion is that the form in which the hypothesis is expressed has important implications for the analysis. If the null hypothesis is nondirectional, the statistical analysis will employ a **two-tailed test of significance**, whereas, if it is directional, the analysis will employ a **one-tailed test**. Since a one-tailed test is more likely to yield a significant result than a two-tailed test, one should always formulate a directional null hypothesis if it is appropriate to specify a direction. In some studies, however, one may not know the direction in which the difference will go, thus necessitating a nondirectional null hypothesis and subsequently the use of less powerful, two-tailed significance tests.

Often, moreover, the way the hypothesis is expressed has important implications for how the study is actually designed. This is why the hypothesis must be quantitatively stated before the study design can be determined (see Step 7).

STEP 6: ANTICIPATE ERROR AND BIAS

Another set of issues that must be explored before determining the study design is the possibility that the results of the study might be rendered inaccurate or misleading by certain types of error or bias that will occur in the data when they are collected. All scientific studies are subject to error and bias, no matter how well designed or carried out. Poorly designed studies, however, are usually more seriously affected, and these distorting influences may invalidate the results and render a study useless and unpublishable. To minimize the occurrence of error or bias in a study, it is crucial to anticipate the types of error or bias that might occur before the study design is determined so that the study may be designed in a way that will minimize the distorting effects of error or bias or allow the investigator to control for them in the statistical analysis.

There are basically four types of error or bias in research studies (Table 6). These are sampling error, selection bias, information bias, and confounding. Although there is a highly developed system for anticipating, avoiding, and testing for sampling error (e.g., sample size calculations and statistical significance testing), the other three types of bias are often more difficult to detect and control.

Suffice it to say that the investigator must anticipate the possibility that biases might be present in data to be collected and take steps in the design of the study to avoid them or in the analysis to control for them. Moreover, the error produced by these types of error and bias in the final results can go in either direction. They can lead to errors in the results that would cause one to conclude erroneously that there is an association (e.g., a difference between groups) when, in fact, there is not (a **Type I error**) or to conclude erroneously that there is not an association when in fact there is (a **Type II error**).

Sampling error is defined as a distortion in the estimate of an association between two variables, resulting from chance variation in the selection of the sample. It usually occurs when the study sample is too small and differences between the comparative groups result from purely random variation. As noted above, this source of error can be minimized by adjusting the sample size in the planning phase of the study (see Step 8). After a study is completed, one can analyze the results to determine the probability that the findings were attributable to a sampling error.

Specifically, if the study came out with a positive finding (the two comparative groups were different on the outcome variable), a statistical significance test can be performed to obtain a **p value** that expresses the probability that the difference occurred by chance alone (due to too small a sample size). If, conversely, the study came out with a negative finding (the two comparative groups were *not* different on the outcome variable), a statistical test can be performed to calculate the **beta probability,** which expresses the probability that the failure to find a difference occurred by chance alone (due to too small a sample size to detect a difference).

In assessing sampling error, the p value is used in a study with a positive outcome to estimate the probability that a Type I error occurred and the beta probability is used in a negative study to estimate the probability that a Type II error occurred.

Selection bias is defined as a distortion in the estimate of an association between two variables, resulting from the manner in which subjects were selected for the study sample. For example, if an investigator asked for volunteers for a study on the causes of lung cancer, it is possible that smokers with longstanding cough who are concerned about lung cancer might be less likely to volunteer for the study than smokers without symptoms. If the smokers who volunteered are compared with nonsmoker volunteers, it is likely that the risk due to smoking will be underestimated because of a selection bias. This would only be known if the investigator anticipated this possibility and included in the project a pilot study to compare the smoker volunteers with smokers in the general population. Unless this is anticipated, the selection bias would lead to an erroneous conclusion.

Table 6. *The 4 types of error or bias in research studies*

Sampling error

A distortion in the estimate of an association between 2 variables, resulting from chance variation in the selection of the sample. It usually occurs when the study sample is too small.

Selection bias

A distortion in the estimate of an association between 2 variables, resulting from the manner in which subjects were selected for the study sample.

Information bias

A distortion in the estimate of an association between 2 variables, resulting from measurement error or misclassification of subjects.

Confounding

A misleading (spurious) association that results when the causal effect of an independent variable on a dependent variable is inflated (or deflated) in a particular set of data by the presence of a third causal variable that is colinked with both the independent variable and the dependent variable.

Information bias is defined as a distortion in the estimate of an association between two variables, resulting from measurement error or misclassification of the subjects, when the error or misclassification is different in the comparative groups. For example, in a study of the dietary risk factors for coronary artery disease, patients with the disease might be more likely to be concerned about the fat content of their diets and might therefore be more likely to record the consumption of fatty foods than would patients without the disease. This might result in an exaggerated estimate of the effect of dietary fat on coronary artery disease due to an error in the way the information was collected. As with selection bias, the potential for information bias must be anticipated and, if a likely possibility, it must be controlled for, if possible, in the analysis of the study.

Confounding is defined as a misleading (spurious) association (Line A—B in Fig. 1) that results when the causal effect of an independent variable (A) on a dependent variable (B) is inflated (or deflated) in a particular set of data by the presence of a third causal variable (C) that is colinked with both the independent variable (A) and the dependent variable (B).

For example, several early studies found that people who drank more than four cups of coffee per day had a higher rate of myocardial infarctions than did people who did not drink coffee. In Fig. 3, coffee drinking would be represented by A and myocardial infarction risk by B. Upon further study, however, it was found that coffee drinking (A) and cigarette smoking (C) were closely linked (dotted line in Fig. 3); coffee drinkers are more likely to smoke than are people who do not drink coffee. Since smoking (C) is known to be a causal factor in outcomes of coronary artery disease (B) and is also associated with coffee drinking (A), it was identified as a potential confounding variable in the analysis. When the analysis was repeated controlling for cigarette smoking, coffee drinking was found not to be associated with myocardial infarction either in smokers or in nonsmokers.

Notice that confounding is different from sampling error, selection bias, and information bias; like the latter two, however, it can only be identified by the anticipations of one who is familiar with the subject matter. Therefore, before finalizing the study design, the investigator must think deeply about the types of error and bias that are likely to be encountered and discuss the possibilities with colleagues to be sure they will be considered in the design and analysis. It is far preferable to think of them at this point, while something can be done, than to learn about them from the anonymous reviewer after the scientific manuscript has been rejected.

STEP 7: DEVELOP THE STUDY DESIGN

After exploring the issues raised in the first six steps, the investigator is ready to develop the strategic design of the study. It is often tempting to decide on the study design earlier in the planning process, but this should be avoided because the main function of the study design is to address the issues raised in the first six steps. In practice, however, it is common to start with a tentative study design and alter it as the first six steps are completed, but the design must not be finalized until the first six steps are completed.

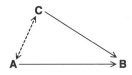

FIG. 1 Schematic diagram of confounding in a set of data from a clinical research project. **A:** The suspected causal factor (coffee drinking). **B:** The disease (heart attacks). **C:** A confounding variable (cigarette smoking). **Solid arrow**; a suspected causal association. **Dashed, double-headed arrow**; a noncausal colinkage.

The Purposes of Studies

In developing the most appropriate design for a study, it is important to identify consciously the purpose of the study. As suggested in Table 7, the purpose of the study often determines the most useful study design.

Generally, the purposes of studies can be divided into descriptive, hypothesis-generating, and hypothesis-testing. In **descriptive studies** the purpose is simply to describe the frequency or magnitude of some event or disease. These studies generally utilize a survey design, almost always utilizing a statistical or convenience sample (see Step 4). If the study's purpose is **hypothesis-generating,** to raise hypotheses for more definitive testing in later studies, one usually relies on a "quick and dirty" observational study, most often of a cohort or case-control design (see below). For the more definitive **hypothesis-testing** purpose, experimental studies (prospective clinical trials) or observational studies of a cohort or case-control design can be used, although if used for hypothesis testing, observational studies must employ extensive design features to avoid or control for bias.

Important Study Designs

Study designs can be divided into three main types: surveys, experiments, and observational (epidemiological, quasi-experimental) studies. The **survey study design** is usually used for studies with descriptive purposes. It involves measuring a set of parameters in one pass through a population or sample of subjects. It is usually performed with a carefully developed and pretested questionnaire and may be administered by mail, by self-administered written format, or by personal interview. This type of study design is most effective for estimating the frequency or magnitude of parameters. It may also be used for measuring associations between variables, although it is usually less satisfactory than other study designs for this purpose.

Most often, surveys are performed in samples of a target universe using one of the many well-described statistical sampling techniques, for example, a simple random sample, a stratified random sample, or a cluster sample. The most common problem of surveys is incomplete response from those surveyed. Since nonrespondents are usually quite different from those who respond, high rates of nonresponse often produce biased results. Consequently, the investigator must often undertake vigorous, repetitive interventions, such as mail or telephone reminders, to obtain the highest possible response. When response rates are low, it is advisable to contact a random sample of the nonrespondents

Table 7. *Relationship between the purpose and the design of research studies*

Purpose	General Design Type Most Often Used
Descriptive	Survey, usually utilizing a statistical sample
Hypothesis-generating	Cross-sectional survey or "quick and dirty" cohort or case-control study
Hypothesis-testing	Experiment (clinical trial) if random assignment is feasible and ethical
	or
	Observational study, often a cohort or case-control design, employing extensive design features to avoid or control for bias, but more elaborate designs are sometimes used.

and obtain enough information to compare with the respondents and estimate the amount of bias due to nonresponse. Sometimes data from prior surveys or alternative data sources can provide enough information for estimating the magnitude of the bias without having to contact a sample of the nonrespondents.

The **experimental study designs** provide a powerful means of testing causal hypotheses in circumstances where treatments or risk factors can be assigned to patients or experimental animals by the investigator. The feature that distinguishes an experimental design from surveys and observational studies is that the treatment or risk factor is assigned by the investigator. Usually, the assignment is randomly determined using a system of random numbers, and ideally both the investigator and the subjects are unaware of which groups the subjects were assigned to (the so-called "double-blind design"). Three of the most commonly used experimental designs—the simple experiment, the repeated measures design, and the repeated measures with crossover design—are portrayed pictorially in Fig. 2 and are explained below.

Most commonly, experimental subjects are randomly assigned to treatment and control (or placebo) groups. The treatment is administered to those in the treatment group, and no treatment (or a placebo) is administered to the control group. Both groups are then followed with identical measurement procedures to determine the number of outcome events in each group. This basic experimental design, referred to as a **simple experiment,** is often varied according to the circumstances of the study.

For example, if the investigator expects a great deal of baseline variation in the outcome measurement, a **repeated measures design** is often used. In this design, two (or more) measurements are performed in all subjects in both the experimental and the control groups, one before the intervention with the treatment or placebo and the second after the intervention has had time to exert its effect. In this design, each patient serves as his or her own control to eliminate the effects of the wide variation in the outcome event. It is important to note that the simple experiment and the repeated measures design require different approaches to the statistical analysis.

For populations involving extreme variation in the outcome event among the subjects, a **crossover component** can be added to the repeated measures design. Under this plan, after completing the repeated measures study, the experiment is repeated in the same experimental and control subjects except that the groups are switched; the treatment is now administered to the control subjects and the placebo to the experimental subjects, and the outcome event is measured again after the treatment has had time to work. When studying interventions such as pharmaceutical agents, whose duration of action is prolonged, it may be necessary to wait for an appropriate time between the first and second stages of the crossover to allow the effects of the treatment to wash out of the subjects. Still different analytical techniques are used to analyze crossover studies.

Observational study designs, also called epidemiological studies or quasi-experiments, are useful in circumstances where experiments are either infeasible or unethical. Although most investigators would prefer to perform experiments, many of the most interesting and pressing clinical issues are not amenable to experimentation and can only be addressed by observational studies. The distinguishing feature of observational studies is that the determination of who receives the treatment or risk factor is not under the control of the investigator. Instead, the investigator measures and analyzes the natural occurrence of independent and dependent variables and performs statistical analyses to obtain the most powerful causal inference possible from the experience.

Simple experiment:	R		X	O			
	R			O			
Repeated measures:	R	O	X	O			
	R	O		O			
Repeated measures with crossover:	R	O	X	O		O	
	R	O		O		X	O

FIG. 2. Strategy diagrams showing the differences among the three most common experimental study designs. **R,** random assignment of patients; **X,** intervention with an experimental treatment; **O,** a period of observation in which the outcome event (dependent variable) is measured.

Observational studies are usually performed in one of two designs: cohort studies or case-control studies (Table 8). In a **cohort study** the subjects are selected on the basis of whether they are exposed to the risk factor (or treatment) and are then followed to determine which ones get the disease. This design is also called a **follow-up study**. For example, using a cohort study design on the problem of smoking and lung cancer, the investigator would classify people on the basis of whether or not they smoke cigarettes (or the number of pack-years of cigarettes smoked) and then would follow the patients forward in time to detect how many cases of lung cancer occurred in each group. Notice that the patients are initially classified according to their cigarette smoking history (the independent variable) and are followed forward in time to measure the occurrence of lung cancer (outcome variable).

In a **case-control study**, sometimes referred to as a "backward study," the design proceeds in the opposite direction from that of a cohort study. The subjects are selected on the basis of whether they have the disease and are then studied to determine which ones had been exposed to the risk factor (or treatment). For example, in using a case-control design to study smoking and lung cancer, the investigator would initially assemble groups of patients with lung cancer and some without lung cancer and would then research back into their medical histories to determine the percentage in each group who smoked cigarettes (or the number of pack-years in each group). Thus, in the case-control design the patients are initially classified on whether or not they have the disease (lung cancer) and are then studied further to determine how many in each group had been smokers.

Although the cohort study design is often seen as the more straightforward and desirable design, both types of study design have a valid and valuable place in clinical research. Generally, cohort studies are used when the outcome under study is relatively frequent in the population to be studied, and case-control designs are usually used for diseases that are rare in the population to be studied or when there is a long latency period between the occurrence of the cause and the disease. This is due to the fact that, for rare diseases or long-latency diseases, cohort studies would have to involve far too many subjects or the subjects would have to be followed for so long between the measurement of the risk factor and the occurrence of the disease that the cohort design would prove far too expensive. For rare or long-latency diseases, it is highly economical, and often just as useful, to identify cases of disease and assemble comparable control groups to carry out case-control studies.

An uncommon but sometimes useful hybrid of the cohort and case-control designs is a **nested case-control** study. The data are initially collected as a typical cohort study (subjects selected on the basis of exposure to the risk factors), but later the investigator selects from the cohort those patients with the disease and a group of controls (with or without matching) for analysis of risk

Table 8. *Definitions of cohort and case-control studies and prospective and retrospective studies*

Cohort study

> The study subjects are selected on the basis of whether they are exposed to the risk factor (or treatment) and are then followed to determine which ones get the disease. Also called a *Followup Study.*

Case-control study

> The study subjects are selected on the basis of whether they have the disease and are then studied to determine which ones had been exposed to the risk factor (or treatment). Also called a *Backward Study.*

Prospective study

> The data on exposures and disease are measured as they occur.

Retrospective study

> The data on exposures and disease are collected long after they occur.

factors, like a case-control study. This can reduce computing costs by reducing the number of patients in the analysis or hold down the costs of recontacting the patients to collect additional risk factor information.

Retrospective versus Prospective Designs

Originally the term **prospective** was used synonymously for cohort studies and **retrospective** was used for case-control studies. In recent years, however, the prospective/retrospective and cohort/case-control distinctions have been disentangled to fit more closely the types of study designs being employed in clinical research. In fact, both cohort and case-control designs can be performed either prospectively or retrospectively, as indicated in Table 9. In current usage, prospective and retrospective are used to designate the time relationship between when the investigator collects the data and when the events occurred. In a prospective study, the events are measured as they occur, whereas in a retrospective study they are measured long after they occur.

In practice, most cohort studies are prospective, and most case-control studies are retrospective (Table 9). Some case-control studies, however, can be prospective. For example, consider a study in which patients with lung cancer are enrolled as they are identified clinically, they are simultaneously paired with a matched control, and risk factors are documented at the same time. This is a case-control study because the patients are initially classified on the basis of the outcome variable (lung cancer), but the information on their cancers is collected prospectively. Likewise, some cohort studies are performed retrospectively. For example, an investigator may assemble a cohort of patients hospitalized in the past and measure both the independent and dependent variables from their hospital medical records (also called a "historical prospective study").

In general, experimental study designs are easier to plan, conduct, and analyze and are less susceptible to error and bias than are observational studies. Observational studies, however, are often less expensive to perform than are experimental studies and may represent the only feasible alternative when experimental designs are infeasible or unethical. In general, a high degree of expertise in epidemiological methods, statistical techniques, and computing skill is required to perform observational studies well. This is because, when randomization is not possible, the investigator must go to much greater lengths to control for the types of error and bias that are predictably present in observational data. On the other hand, error and bias can also creep into experimental designs, making it desirable to obtain the assistance of a qualified statistician in designing and analyzing all clinical studies.

STEP 8: ESTIMATE THE SAMPLE SIZE NEEDED

Determination of the optimal sample size for a study is a critical feature of the design. If too few subjects are chosen, the study is likely to fall prey to sampling error, ending in either a Type I or a Type II error (see Step 6 above). On the other hand, selecting too many subjects may increase the cost of the study beyond the financial resources available. To avoid either extreme, the investigator must predict the optimal number and use that in selecting the subjects for study.

To select the optimal sample size, the investigator must make an **educated guess** about the number of subjects who will be needed to obtain a valid test of the hypothesis under study. To do this, one must simply predict what numerical results will be obtained at the end of the study and then work backward to the sample size needed to test for statistical significance. New investigators are often uncomfortable with determining the sample size on the basis of an educated guess. What if the guess is wrong? Unfortunately there is no way of guaranteeing an adequate sample size. Instead, a great deal of effort must be put into making the best educated guess possible for determining the sample size.

Table 9. *The relationship between the cohort/case-control and prospective/ retrospective designations in clinical research*

	Cohort	Case-Control
Prospective	*common*	*uncommon*
Retrospective	*uncommon[a]*	*common*

[a]Also called an "historical prospective" design; in this design the researcher analyzes data from records compiled "prospectively," long in the past (e.g., hospital medical records).

For instance, one may find data in published studies or perform pilot studies to obtain more reliable guesses of the parameters.

In most instances, new investigators should consult a qualified statistician to assist in estimating the required sample size, since the exact method depends on the type of study design selected (see Step 7). In general, though, for each type of study design, there are only a small number of parameters that must be measured, estimated, or guessed at to form the basis for estimating the optimal sample size. For example, in a simple survey for estimating the frequency of some clinical parameter in a population, one simply needs to know the estimated frequency (percentage) at which the parameter will be found in the population and then specify how far off the estimate can be from the true value due to sampling variation (e.g., the desired width of the confidence intervals around the estimate) and the degree of assurance that the estimate will be made with a specified level of precision (the alpha and beta probabilities). By making a best guess at these parameters, the investigator provides all the information needed for the statistician to calculate the sample size for the study. With experience, one can often arrive at a satisfactory sample size estimate by entering the required parameter estimates into the sample size program of one of the standard statistical packages for personal computers.

STEP 9: WRITE A RESEARCH PROTOCOL FOR ALL COLLABORATORS TO REVIEW

As with writing down the specific objectives of the study, it is crucial that the investigator write a description of the study plan, including the issues covered in the previous steps, before beginning work on the project. By writing the protocol the investigator clarifies the exact intent and details of the proposed plan. In the absence of a written protocol, crucial details or concepts will be confused, vague, or frankly conflicting, and many of these problems will not be noticed. Most become glaringly obvious when they are written. A written description of the study is also needed for grant applications and proposals to an institutional review board.

Particularly when collaborating with other investigators, it is immensely helpful to pass a draft protocol among the collaborators to "smoke out" issues on which there was unsuspected disagreement. It is far better that these issues be clarified early in the design phase rather than after the data are collected when it is too late to correct them.

It is also useful to designate assignments for the time-consuming parts of the work entailed in the protocol and to assign at least a tentative authorship list for publications resulting from the study. Often authorship can be determined without disagreement before the work is done, and collaborators will tend to participate to the degree that they are to be recognized as coauthors. If authorship is left until the manuscript is written, serious, sometimes bitter, disagreements may arise.

By writing down the protocol at this point in the design process and passing it among the collaborating investigators, the basic objectives and design can be agreed upon. Subsequently, as further steps are completed, the protocol can be extended to include the additional elements of the design. In this way, all collaborators can remain current on the state of the design at any time.

STEP 10: PLAN THE DATA COLLECTION PROCESS

It is important to plan the data collection process in great detail to ensure the accuracy of the measurements of the independent variables, the dependent variables, and the extraneous variables. Often the plans represent a detailed description of the laboratory methods or survey questionnaires; these should be described in step-by-step detail to ensure that all steps are explicit ahead of time. Forms used to record the data should also be developed and, if appropriate, tested for accuracy and clarity in a pilot study ahead of the main data collection process. If the accuracy of the data collection methods has not already been ascertained in prior studies, the investigators should undertake validation studies to measure the validity and/or the reproducibility of the measurements.

Where a "gold standard" (an alternative method known to be highly accurate) exists, the new laboratory method should be compared with it in a pilot study to measure the **validity** of the new method. Measurements of validity result in estimating four parameters: sensitivity, specificity, the predictive value of a positive, and the predictive value of a negative. As shown in Table 10, the

sensitivity is the probability that, if the patient has the disease, the new method will be positive. The **specificity** is the probability that, if the patient does not have the disease, the test will be negative. The **predictive value of a positive** is the probability that, if the test is positive, the patient will have the disease. The **predictive value of a negative** is the probability that, if the test is negative, the patient will not have the disease. In general, the sensitivity and specificity are most useful when doing scientific studies, and the predictive value parameters are most useful when using a screening test in the care of an individual patient.

When no "gold standard" method exists, one can at least measure the reproducibility, or **reliability**, of the new measurement method. In studies where a method is to be used by a number of data collectors, the pilot study generally involves having 2 to 5 representative data collectors use it to make independent measurements on a moderate number of subjects, usually 15 to 25. The level of agreement among the simultaneous "raters" is expressed with a statistic called Cohen's kappa, which measures on a scale of 0 to 1 the level of agreement above that expected by chance alone.

STEP 11: MANAGE AND MONITOR DATA COLLECTION

The difficulty of collecting accurate clinical data is often underestimated by new investigators. In the words of one veteran mentor of young researchers, "Data doesn't collect itself." The perturbing influences that would introduce error and bias into an otherwise marvelous study design are legion in the everyday world of clinical research. To overcome these influences and collect valid observations, with the beginning of the data collection phase the investigator must undergo a transformation from intellectual designer into a hard-nosed, uncompromising though inspiring task master, ensuring that all aspects of the protocol are strictly adhered to.

Most importantly, the investigator must learn to distinguish between what is scientifically right and what is easy. Compromise often results in misclassification of subjects. If the misclassification is merely random, it reduces the chance of finding a significant difference. If it is systematic and related to the hypothesis under study, it constitutes a bias and will distort the study's results. For example, in prospective clinical trials of new treatments, a natural tension exists between the clinical investigator and the experimental subjects' personal physicians. In some studies there is a tendency for some personal physicians to want to get certain patients, say, those with no hope of cure with present treatments, into the experimental arm rather than the placebo group. If the randomized protocol has been approved by an institutional review board and true informed consent has been obtained, the investigator must either take steps

Table 10. *Analysis of data collected in a pilot study to determine the validity of a new method of measurement in comparison with an established method known to be highly accurate (a "gold standard")*

		Gold Standard		
		Disease	No disease	
Result from New Test	Pos	a	b	a/a+b = PVP
	Neg	c	d	c/c+c = PVN
		a/a+c= sensitivity	b/b+d= specificity	

PVP = predictive value of a positive.   **PVN** = predictive value of a negative.

to prevent the random assignment protocol from being subverted or abandon the study.

In laboratory studies or small epidemiological studies, the volume of data collection work is often small enough for the investigator to perform it alone or with one or two assistants. When using an assistant, it is wise for the investigator to know more about the measurement methods than the assistant and to use the assistant as an extension of his or her hands rather than entirely delegating the work. In more extensive studies where the amount of work requires a larger data collection staff, the investigator must become a **professional manager,** that is, one who is skilled in management science. This requires knowledge of project phasing, scheduling, and monitoring; personnel screening, hiring, and supervision; effective leadership styles; time management; and financial and budgetary management, to name but a few of the required skills. While these may come easy to some, most young investigators can substantially hone their management skills by reading and taking courses in management.

Particularly useful tools for planning and managing the data collection process are the **PERT** (program evaluation and review technique) charts and **Gantt** charts. Both utilize charts showing the various tasks, or phases, on a time scale. PERT charts display the various tasks as round "nodes" connected by lines between related tasks, whereas Gantt charts display the tasks as rectangular boxes arranged on a time scale and extending from the beginning to the time of completion of the task. An example of a Gantt chart for completing a complex three-day metabolic study on patients enrolled in a clinical research study is shown in Fig. 3. PERT and Gantt charts are invaluable not only for carrying out work on an efficient schedule but also for ensuring that projects are completed within an allotted time frame. The latter is often crucial in certain contract research that calls for adherence to deadlines.

As data collection progresses, the investigator must continue to monitor the accuracy of the data to ensure that the assistants do not become lax in the accuracy of their work. This monitoring function may be as simple as periodically looking over the shoulder of a laboratory technician or as extensive as having a certain percentage of the subjects studied independently by two or more of the data collectors as an in-line check on the reliability of the measurements.

STEP 12: MANAGE THE DATABASE

The database is the quantitative record of the values of the dependent, independent, and extraneous variables measured on all of the subjects in the study. In small clinical studies involving only a few patients, the data can often be effectively managed solely on paper forms or by recording in notebooks. Larger clinical studies, however, require storing the data in a computer. Moderate size databases can often be managed by the investigator using one of the commercially available database management software packages. The management of large databases may require the assistance of a staff of trained database programmers.

The larger the size of the database the more important it is to set up procedures for accounting for the data collection forms to avoid losing them, entering and editing the data to minimize data entry errors, and backing up the database to avoid losing it in an archiving accident. Each dataset should be fully documented in a notebook containing the data collection form, the record layout showing the column assignments of all the variables in the raw data file, the list of variables and their definitions and valid codes, the definitions of new variables created by computer programs after data collection, and the pertinent history of the database, such as the dates of the beginning and ending of data collection and of any changes in variable definitions. Although database documentation often seems superfluous at the beginning of a project, it usually proves essential later in the analysis phase when memories of the many complex features and decisions of the data collection phase begin to fade and become blurred. Often simply keeping a three-ring notebook with appropriate dividers to file key pieces of documentation saves countless hours or hopeless confusion later in the study.

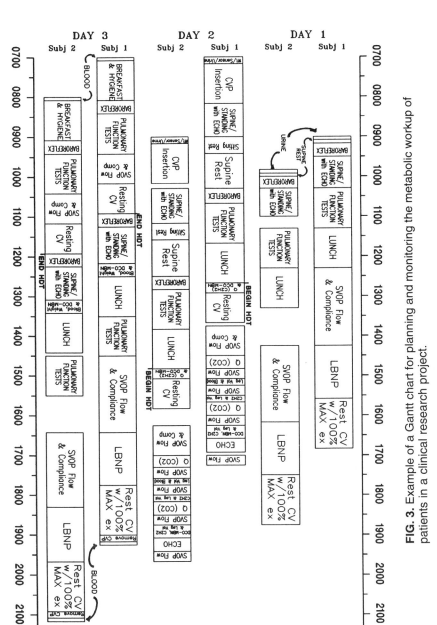

FIG. 3. Example of a Gantt chart for planning and monitoring the metabolic workup of patients in a clinical research project.

STEP 13: ANALYZE THE RESULTS INTO TABLES AND GRAPHS

While new investigators often tend to become preoccupied with statistical tests of significance, the real heart of analyzing the data from a clinical research project is conceiving of and producing the tables and graphs that most effectively test the hypothesis and describe the results. Ideally, the most important tables and graphs are conceived ahead of time in the design phase, but in most studies some amount of additional analysis is necessary to find the most enlightening way of displaying the results so that they will convey the findings most powerfully to the journal reader. For example, exploratory analysis is often essential for testing the normality of distributions of continuous variables, identifying extreme observations ("outliers") that would bias the calculation of means and perturb statistical tests, testing for confounding variables, and performing poststratified analyses to control for biasing factors. Much of this work depends on the content of the database and cannot be entirely anticipated ahead of time.

Almost always the analysis of the research database is done with one of the many computerized statistical packages. At first the investigator should work closely with a statistician to ensure that the analyses are done correctly and completely. After more experience, the investigator may assume progressively more of the analytic responsibilities to get more of his or her intuition into the analytic process. Even the most experienced researchers, however, continue consulting qualified statisticians on important aspects of their analyses and ask them to review draft manuscripts from a statistical perspective before submitting them to scientific journals. Since well-qualified statisticians often have preferred methods and approaches to analysis, it is wise to involve the statistician, who will assist with the analysis of the results, in the design phase of the project.

STEP 14: TEST THE HYPOTHESIS WITH THE CORRECT STATISTICAL TESTS

Early in the design phase, it is important that the investigator anticipate the statistical test(s) that is to be applied to the final results. Even though the statistical process will ultimately prove more extensive, the basic statistical approach should be thought through early in the design.

Although the art of statistical testing is often seen as a mystical, and sometimes unfathomable, process for new investigators, the basic approach for choosing the right statistical test is really quite simple. To choose the right statistical test in the majority of circumstances, the investigator must ask four simple questions (Table 11). The answers to these four questions will determine the most appropriate statistical test in the majority of instances.

First, one asks, "What are the variables being compared?" To answer this question, the investigator identifies the independent variable(s) and the outcome variable that are to be compared in the central hypothesis test at the end of the study. (In many studies there will be extraneous or confounding variables to be analyzed as well, but these go beyond the elemental approach being presented here.)

Second, when the variables are identified, the investigator asks, "What is the form of these variables?" and identifies what type of variable each is. Is each a categorical, dichotomous variable; a categorical, multicategoried, nominal variable; a categorical, multicategoried, ordered variable; or a continuous (or interval) variable?

Third, if the outcome variable is continuous, the investigator asks, "Does it meet the normality assumption?" This question is answered by graphing the distribution of the outcome variable in the population to be studied. This can

Table 11. *The 4 practical questions to ask in determining the most appropriate method of statistical analysis and test of statistical significance*[a]

1. What are the independent and dependent variables?

2. What type of variables are they?

    Categorical, dichotomous
    Categorical, multicategoried, nominal
    Categorical, multicategoried, ordered
    Continuous (or interval)

3. If the outcome variable is continuous, does it meet the Normality Assumption?

4. Are the observations independent or paired?[b]

[a] The answers to these questions will allow selection of appropriate statistical tests in the majority of instances, but confidence in the selection requires ample research experience or consultation with a statistician.

[b] Paired observations are most often found in repeated measures experiments and matched case-control studies.

often be done by data obtained on this or a similar population from previous studies or from the literature, or the investigator may wish to perform a pilot study to estimate the distribution.

Finally, the investigator asks, "Are the comparison groups independent or paired?" In simple experiments, most cohort studies, and some case-control studies, the observations on the study subjects are independent of one another, and the answer to the question is "no." In repeated measures experimental designs and in matched case-control studies, the observations on the subjects are paired, in which case the answer to the question is "yes."

Tables 12 and 13 indicate the usual analysis strategy, the measure of association used, and the test of statistical significance that is most commonly used given the answers to these four questions. In the majority of clinical studies, the outcome variable is either a dichotomous (two-category) categorical variable (portrayed in Table 12) or a continuous (or interval) variable (portrayed in Table 13). In each of these two instances, the independent variable can be any of the four types of variables, and these are portrayed in the first column of each table. For each of the resulting rows of the two tables, the usual type of statistical analysis performed, the most useful measures of the association between the independent and dependent variables, and the usual tests of statistical significance (to estimate the probability of a Type I sampling error) are given.

Table 12. *Simplified Scheme for choosing statistical tests for two-category (dichotomous) outcome variables*

Group/Predictor variable	Outcome variable	Nonparametric Procedures		
		Analysis	Measure of association	Test of statistical significance
Two-category (dichotomous)	Two-category	2 x 2 contingency table	Relative risk (odds ratio)	Chi-square test Fisher's exact test 95% confidence interval of the relative risk McNemar's test [a]
Multi-category, Nominal	Two-category	n x 2 contingency table	Uncertainty Coefficient	Chi-square test
Multi-category, Ordered	Two-category	n x 2 contingency table	Goodman-Kruskal gamma	Chi-square test Chi-square test for trend
Continuous	Two-category	Usually recode independent variable to categories and analyze it by the appropriate method above, or use logistic regression analysis.		

[a] Used for paired observations.

For example, most commonly in cohort and case-control studies, both the independent and dependent variables are **dichotomous (two-categoried) categorical** variables. Therefore, look at Table 12, which deals with dichotomous categorical dependent variables. The appropriate analysis, shown on the first row, is a 2 x 2 contingency table, the relative risk is the most appropriate measure of association between the two variables, and the usual significance test is a *p* value calculated with the chi-square test or Fisher's exact test. Increasingly, the 95% confidence intervals of the relative risk are being used in place of the *p* value from the chi-square test or Fisher's exact test. If the observations were paired, as in a repeated measures experimental design or a matched case-control study, McNemar's test is used instead of the chi-square or Fisher's exact test.

When the dependent variable is **continuous** (or interval) data, consult Table 13, which portrays the options for continuous outcome variables. The most appropriate analyses must also consider whether the continuous outcome variable is normally distributed or not, indicated in the third column in the table. If the continuous outcome variable is normally distributed, the investigator can use a powerful set of tests that compare the mean value of the outcome variable in the experimental and control groups. (Tests that compare the means of continuous variables are referred to by the cryptic term **parametric tests.**) The measure of the association between the two comparison groups is usually the difference between the means, and the most commonly used statistical test is Student's *t* test.

If the variables are not continuously distributed, that is, the distribution of the continuous outcome variable is skewed to the right or the left, the investigator has two choices. One can transform the outcome variable by an appropriate transformation (e.g., taking the logarithm, the square, or the square root of each patient's value) into a nearly normal distribution and then use one of the powerful sets of parametric tests that compare the means. Alternatively, one can use a different set of statistical tests that do not require that the data be normally distributed. (These are referred to as **nonparametric tests.**) Examples of nonparametric tests are Wilcoxon's rank-sum test, or the Mann-Whitney U test, and the median test. These have the advantage of not requiring normality in the continuous outcome variables, but they are generally not quite as likely to show significance (i.e., they generally have slightly less statistical power than the parametric tests). If the observations are paired, the most often used parametric test is the paired *t* test, and the most often used nonparametric test is the signed rank test.

The final end-product of all statistical tests is the *p* **value**. The *p* value is nothing more than the probability (measured from 0 to 1) that the observed difference between the experimental and the control groups occurred by chance alone due to sampling error. When the *p* value is less than 0.05 it is generally

Table 13. *Simplified scheme for choosing statistical tests for continuous outcome variables.*

Group/Predicator variable	Outcome Variable	Normality assumption satisfied	Parametric Procedures			Nonparametric
			Analysis	Measure of Association	Test of Statistical Significance	Test of Statistical Significance
Two-category (dichotomous)	Continuous	Yes	Compare means	Difference between means	Student's t test Paired t test*	(Not Needed)
		No	Transform the data and compare means	Difference between transformed means	Student's t test Paired t test*	(Not Needed)
			Or use Nonparametric test			Mann-Whitney U test Rank-Sum test Median test Signed rank test [a]
Multi-category, Nominal	Continuous	Yes	Compare means by ANOVA	Difference between means	F-test	(Not Needed)
		No	Transform the data and compare means by ANOVA	Difference between transformed means	F-test	(Not Needed)
			Or use Nonparametric tests	Difference between medians		Kruskal-Wallis non-parametric ANOVA

Table 13. (contd.) *Simplified scheme for choosing statistical tests for continuous outcome variables.*

Multi-category, Ordered	Continuous	Yes	Compare means by ANOVA	Difference between means	F-test	(Not Needed)
		No	Transform the data and compare means by ANOVA	Difference between transformed means	F-test	(Not Needed)
			Or use Nonparametric tests	Difference between medians		Kruskal-Wallis non-parametric ANOVA
Continuous	Continuous	Yes	Correlation or regression analysis	Pearson's r or regression coefficient	F-test	(Not Needed)
		No	Transform the data and do correlation or regression	Difference between transformed means	F-test	(Not Needed)
			Or use Nonparametric tests	Spearman's r medians		Spearman rank order correlation

[a] Used for paired observations.

77

conceded that sampling error has been ruled out as an explanation for the difference.

It is important to know, however, that in many studies the critical value of p that determines statistical significance might vary. In some studies an investigator might require a p value of 0.001 for statistical significance, particularly if many significance tests were being done in a row. In other studies, one might accept a p value as high as 0.10 as statistically significant, for example, if there were disastrous consequences for making a Type II error.

It is also important to realize that the p value deals only with sampling error and does not give any information as to the likelihood of the other types of bias (selection bias, information bias, and confounding). These can only be assessed by thinking of the likely biases and doing further statistical analyses to determine whether they account for the differences found.

STEP 15: GENERATE ADDITIONAL TABLES AND GRAPHS TO EXPLAIN THE FINDINGS

After the main test is performed, the investigator or the consulting statistician will generally perform additional analyses to elaborate on the findings. For example, after finding an association between the independent and dependent variables, it might be desirable to perform a test to demonstrate a dose-response relationship or to repeat the main analysis controlling for extraneous variables. These additional analyses should be anticipated in the design phase so that the variables will be appropriately coded and the sample sizes will be adequate for them.

STEP 16: PUBLISH THE RESULTS IN A SCIENTIFIC JOURNAL

Finally, the end-product of a successful study is the publication of an article in a scientific journal. Remember, if a study is not published, it was never done. Successful writing for scientific journals is an art form that must be acquired through study and practice. It is different from other styles of writing.

One should always decide on a specific journal before starting to write a scientific article, consult the "Information for Authors" page that appears in most of the journals, customize the article according to those instructions, and photocopy several articles from recent issues of the journal to serve as models.

Generally, a good scientific article presents no more than four or five main points that are the key findings in the results section. These should be illustrated by tables and graphs in nearly final form before sitting down to write. The writing process goes much smoother if the tables and graphs are completely laid out and the results are written to describe and relate to them.

Clear writing requires an outline, and papers written without an outline are often disorganized. After the initial draft is made, it should be revised over and over again and passed among colleagues for critical review and revision.

CONCLUSION

Designing clinical research projects is a creative and rigorous process that requires attention to a large number of details, each of which can determine the success or failure of the project. For the planning and execution of projects to be successful, the investigator must be fully aware of the many aspects that must be planned so that all are addressed as early as possible in the research process. The steps outlined in this chapter provide a road map to give new investigators a framework and a checklist for the issues that they must address in planning their research projects. Proficiency in designing research requires study of more detailed references on these subjects and the guidance of experienced colleagues and mentors.

ADDITIONAL READING

1. Fleiss, J.L. (1986): *The Design and Analysis of Clinical Experiments.* John Wiley & Sons, New York.
2. Friedman, L.M., Furberg, C.D., and DeMets, D.L. (1981): *Fundamentals of Clinical Trials.* John Wright PSG, Boston.
3. Graziano, A.M. and Raulin, M.L. (1989):*Research Methods: A Process of Inquiry.* Harper & Row, Publishers, New York.
4. Hennekens, C.H. and Buring, J.E. (1987): *Epidemiology in Medicine.* Little, Brown and Company, Boston.
5. Marks, R.G. (1982): *Designing a Research Project: The Basics of Biomedical Research Methodology.* Lifetime Learning Publications, Belmont, CA.
6. Miettinen, O.S. (1985): *Theoretical Epidemiology: Principles of Occurrence Research in Medicine.* Delmar Publishers, Albany, NY.
7. Murrell, G., Huang, C., Ellis, H., and Langdon, D. (1990): *Research in Medicine: A Guide to Writing a Thesis in the Medical Sciences.* Cambridge University Press, New York.
8. Payton, O.D. (1988): *Research: The Validation of Clinical Practice. 2nd ed.* F.A. Davis Company, Philadelphia.
9. Rothman, K.J. (1986): *Modern Epidemiology.* Little, Brown and Company, Boston.

10. Schlesselman, J.J. (1982): *Case-control Studies: Design, Conduct, Analysis.* Oxford University Press, New York.
11. Stein, F. (1989): *Anatomy of Clinical Research: An Introduction to Scientific Inquiry in Medicine, Rehabilitation and Related Health Professions.* Slack, Thorofare, NJ.
12. Troidl, H., Spitzer, W.O., McPeek, B., Mulder, D.S., McKneally, M.F., Wechsler, A.S., and Balch, C.M. (1991): *Principles and Practice of Research: Strategies for Surgical Investigators. 2nd ed.* Springer-Verlag, New York.

6

Statistical Considerations for Clinical Research

Joan S. Reisch, Ph.D.

Academic Computing Services, University of Texas Southwestern Medical Center at Dallas, Dallas, Texas 75235-9066

Statistical principles influence the planning of a clinical study, its execution, and the interpretation of the results. This chapter focuses primarily on these principles in the belief that the clinical investigator has a variety of resources for carrying out the details of the appropriate statistical analyses, including consultation with statisticians and access to appropriate computer software and hardware resources.

For the investigator interested in more detail, there are excellent references for the design of clinical trials. The texts by Pocock (15) and by Friedman et al. (8) are excellent overviews with many practical suggestions. Meinert (13) and Spilker (18) provide in-depth treatments of the design, execution, management, and reporting principles for clinical trials.

The purpose of this chapter is not to cover the mathematics of the statistical analysis but to consider the principles that influence the statistical analysis in a well-done clinical investigation.

SPECIFIC RESEARCH QUESTIONS

In Chapter 5, steps in designing clinical research are covered. As Dr. Haley states, the basis for successful clinical research is the idea for the study. The idea may come from one or a combination of sources. It may occur while reading the latest research reports, attending a scientific meeting, treating patients, or discussing research with colleagues.

With the idea(s) in mind, a review of the scientific literature may reveal results, techniques, and further ideas to explore with colleagues. These discussions may help refine the primary and secondary research questions on which the study will focus. The primary and secondary research questions should be formulated before collecting any data. The methods of assessment—laboratory, clinical, or psychological—should be chosen and examined for their feasibility early in the design process. If possible, subgroup analyses should be planned in advance.

A primary research question should be specific. For example, a study of a treatment or management method designed to reduce hypertension may require answers to several questions. What is hypertension? How will the treatment effect be measured? Who will be the subjects? Other needed specifications may include the statement of the doses of drug(s) which make up the treatment(s), as well as selection of the endpoints (change in absolute value, percentage of change, reduction to clinically "normal," etc.). Secondary questions might include accompanying changes in high-density lipoproteins (HDLs), LDLs, or very-low-density lipoprotein (VLDL) cholesterol or triglycerides. Subgroup analyses could involve the comparisons of a more severely hypertensive subgroup to one with milder hypertension within each of the treatment or management groups.

Statistical methods are utilized for several purposes: descriptive, relational, and comparative. They can be used to summarize the demographic characteristics of members of a group treated with a diet and exercise regimen; they may assess potential relationships between such measurements as age or clinical status and diastolic blood pressure level. A group managed with diet and exercise may be compared to a group treated with a diuretic, or comparisons may be made within a single group from before to after treatment. If an important endpoint involves mortality, techniques of survival analysis may be employed. Since most studies involve the measurement of several characteristics, rather than just one, multivariate methods may be required for appropriate analysis of results.

POPULATION/SAMPLE

In the planning process the investigator should select the population to which the results will be generalized, referred to as the *target population.* The investigator might ask the following questions in defining the target population: Of what population from a hypertension clinic are the subjects representative? Hypertensive patients in a large city-county hospital? Hypertensive patients in Texas? In the United States? Or in the world?

It would be unusual to be able to study the entire population of interest, so the researcher studies a part of the population, referred to as the *sample.* The technique of selecting study subjects from a target population is called *sampling.* The most desirable sampling method to use involves some random process; the subjects may be selected at random from a population or they may be an arbitrary set of subjects assigned at random to different treatment groups. Randomization reduces the likelihood of bias and provides the basis for the valid application of statistical techniques.

Convenience sampling is another selection procedure. A sample of women encountered at a particular shopping center on a summer weekend day queried about their breast cancer knowledge is a group obtained conveniently. The selection process may introduce bias into the study, and it is difficult to generalize about the target population because the women willing to participate may be representative only of themselves.

Subjects cannot be assigned at random if an investigator's study involves the comparison of a group of subjects with a particular disease to a group of subjects without the disease (but still thought to be comparable in all aspects but the disease). The subjects, however, could be selected at random from each of their respective target populations.

The investigator needs to consider very carefully what sampling method to utilize. A well-done clinical study almost always involves some random component in the sampling procedure. Pocock's text (15) provides examples of randomizing subjects. Assistance with randomization can be obtained by consulting a professional statistician.

Sample sizes can be selected according to statistical principles, and clinical information useful for calculating appropriate sample sizes may be available in the literature. Later in this chapter, sample size criteria are discussed in more detail and examples are given to illustrate the computations.

INCLUSION/EXCLUSION CRITERIA

The investigator defines the required characteristics of the subjects to be studied. The inclusion and exclusion criteria are specific to a particular study. The criteria for selecting (or not selecting) a subject for inclusion should be consistent with the target population(s). Demographic characteristics—age, sex, and race—are usually important. Recent changes in federal research guidelines require an investigator to indicate specific reasons for excluding women or minorities as subjects. Clinical history variables such as previous treatment, family history of a disease, or reaching previous endpoints (e.g., a prior myocardial infarction) may be reasons for inclusion or exclusion in the study. Any contraindications for treatment/management should be listed, including family history and concomitant medical problems. A subject's disease status may be important in the risk-to-benefit ratio for the subject. In studying the treatment of a terminal illness, the subject's life expectancy should be long enough for the subject's potential benefit.

A subject's ability to communicate in English may be a consideration when considerable communication is required in the treatment process or when written instruments are involved. Particular subjects may be known to be erratic in following treatment procedures or in keeping clinic appointments. The researchers could exclude them initially for their assumed or stated inability to comply with study requirements.

Characteristics that might affect the endpoints and that could confound the results should also be considered, measured, and adjusted for in the statistical analysis of results.

COMPARISON (OR CONTROL) GROUP

Good scientific practice calls for a comparison (or control) group to be included in a study of a new treatment or management method. The control treatment may involve no treatment, a treatment with a placebo that is not physically distinguishable from the intervention being studied, or the current standard treatment. The control subjects should be managed in exactly the same manner as the subjects undergoing the treatment under investigation. Then, when the treated and control groups are compared, the results of the treatment can be distinguished from the act of treating.

All potential study subjects must meet the same entry criteria before informed consent is obtained. Then they are assigned to the treatment groups, usually in equal numbers.

Members of the control group are studied concurrently with the treated group so that any conditions of the environment or the care-giving personnel are relatively constant. It has been found that, when results for currently treated subjects are compared to those of subjects assessed earlier (i.e., historical controls), the treatment effect tends to be exaggerated.

If information is available from a comparison group from an earlier time period, the allocation of subjects to the control group may be reduced. The analysis could involve both the randomized and the historical controls, with weight given to the concurrent control group data (15). In a study of subjects with a rare disease (e.g., amyotrophic lateral sclerosis), it may be more justifiable to use historical controls if their clinical information was obtained recently and under similar circumstances.

RANDOMIZATION, STRATIFICATION, AND BLOCKING

In randomizing subjects to a treatment, neither the investigator nor the subject influences the treatment assignment. Random selection or assignment does not guarantee the representativeness of the sample, but it does reduce bias and it is the basis for valid statistical hypothesis testing and the resulting probability (or *p)* values.

The investigator may wish to use stratification, a process that divides subjects into subsets or strata, as a way of making sure that each stratum is represented in the sample and as a way of making the treatment groups comparable at the beginning of the study. Usually, two stratifying factors are the maximum practical.

For example, sex and clinical history could be chosen as the important stratifying factors in the study of treatment of hypertension. If the clinical history strata are the presence or absence of previous treatment, then four strata result: females with and without previous treatment and males with and without previous treatment. Randomization within each stratum will result in proportional (usually) numbers of subjects in each treatment group within each stratum as well as overall. If the investigator wishes to analyze the data for each stratum separately, he or she must plan for sufficient subjects in each stratum.

Another desirable restriction in the treatment assignment process may involve blocking, which results in an equal number of subjects in each treatment or management group within so many multiples of the number of treatments. As an example, blocking in a study comparing two treatments could involve randomizing so that there are three subjects in each treatment group after every set of six subjects is entered. The first six subjects make up the first block, the next six subjects are part of the second, and so forth. The order of treatment assignments is randomized and usually different for each subsequent block. The investigator could choose blocks of four, six, eight, ten, and so forth.

Blocking may be beneficial because many subtle factors that might influence the important outcome measurements may change over time. These factors might include differences in batches of medication, in care-giving or technical personnel, in the environment, or in instrumentation. Within a particular block of subjects, the effects of these external factors tend to be more consistent.

An additional benefit of blocking is that if the study needs to be stopped prematurely because one treatment is obviously superior or harmful, there would be essentially proportional numbers of subjects in each treatment group.

STUDY DESIGN

The study design may involve independent groups, related groups, or a combination of both. In clinical studies, the combination of independent groups studied repeatedly over time is a common design.

Let's look first at a simple design that involves independent groups. Independent samples are those in which each group of subjects receives a different treatment. At least two different treatments are studied, but there may be as many as ten or more different treatment groups. There may be one control group, or even two or three (e.g., no treatment, placebo, and current standard treatment). Measurements are made at a point in time, and the desired comparisons are made to answer the research questions. Each subject belongs to one and only one treatment group.

On the other hand, related samples are those in which the same subjects are evaluated at a minimum of two different points in the course of the study. It is desirable to randomize the order of the treatments the subjects receive. (This is not possible in a study in which the subject is evaluated before and after an intervention.) A design that involves one group of subjects evaluated at two points in time is the simplest example of a repeated measures design.

Pairs of subjects may be matched for relevant characteristics on a one-for-one basis and randomly assigned to treatment groups. The deliberate matching design is a repeated measures design even though different subjects are in each treatment group; the appropriate statistical analysis considers the pairing aspect.

Crossover studies are ones in which a group of subjects undergoes each of the treatments under investigation in random order. In a two-treatment crossover study one-half the subjects get Treatment A first and B second; the other half get Treatment B first and A second. These designs are appropriate in the study of chronic diseases (asthma, arthritis, diabetes, hypertension) in which a "cure" is not expected. An advantage of a crossover study is that the effect, if any, of the order of the interventions can be assessed in addition to the differences between the interventions.

While crossover studies provide for the ultimate matching (the same subject has values for each pair, triplet, etc., of data), an underlying assumption is that the treatments do not have a residual effect. If this is an unreasonable assumption, the investigator should consider a "washout" period between the two treatments. The length of this washout period should exceed the amount of time the treatments are known to have an effect after being stopped. By including a washout period, it is expected that the starting points of both treatments are comparable. The investigator may also consider having a baseline period at the end as well as the beginning of the study.

Most designs in clinical studies involve combinations of these two basic designs: two or more independent groups are evaluated at two or more intervals during the course of the study. These are also repeated measures designs.

THE SCALE OF MEASUREMENT

It is important to know the scale of measurement for treatment and response variables because it influences sample size determination and the choice of appropriate descriptive, relational, and comparative statistical techniques. Scales of measurement can be divided into three categories: (a) nominal or categorical; (b) ordinal or rank order; or (c) continuous (interval or ratio).

Nominal

Using a nominal scale of measurement, a variable is "measured" by counting sample members in a category. Sex is measured on a nominal scale: male or female. In the early days of computing, numerical values were assigned to categories. Thus, sample means could be computed even for arbitrarily assigned values. The "average" sex of a sample equal to 1.23 indicates that there are more members of the sample who are assigned the value of sex equal to 1 than 2.

A descriptive statistic more appropriate than the mean for the variable "sex" is the proportion (or percentage) of males or females in each treatment group or the ratio of males to females. Another is the mode, the most frequently occurring value. Other examples of variables measured on a nominal scale are marital status, ethnic background, diagnostic category, clinical service, and religious affiliation.

Ordinal

For variables measured on an ordinal scale, members of the sample can be ranked in order of magnitude from lowest to highest or from highest to lowest. Results of laboratory tests with values of negative, 1+, 2+, 3+, or 4+ are examples. The median is an appropriate "average" for ordinal measurement; the range is an appropriate measure of variability.

Assessments such as mild, moderate, or severe may seem to be nominal measurements but, in fact, are ordinal because these categories can be ordered and ranks assigned. The numbers, proportions, or percentages for each rank can be reported. Psychological scales with answers such as "Disagree strongly," "Disagree," "No opinion," "Agree," or "Agree strongly" are ordinal in nature.

Continuous

Measurements on a continuous scale take one of two forms: interval or ratio. Both forms of continuous measurement are truly numerical on a mathematical scale that has a constant interval size (e.g., inches, hours, concentration). A measurement on an interval scale has an arbitrary zero point. Examples include time of day and year (e.g. the time of day that a baby is born or when a death occurs), compass directions (location of a tumor in breast cancer), and temperature (Fahrenheit and Celsius but not absolute or Kelvin).

The descriptive statistics and the comparative methods for interval continuous variables are somewhat unique. The techniques for finding the averages of angles or times (even on a 24-hour basis) are not the ordinary means, medians, or modes. Although a range is an appropriate measure of variability, a standard deviation or standard error is not. The text by Zar (20) is remarkable for its inclusion of appropriate statistical descriptive and comparative techniques for treating these data.

More usual continuous variables are ratio variables, which are measured on a numerical scale with constant interval size and a zero point that has physical meaning. Examples include height, weight, elapsed time, change in temperature, duration of illness, serum creatinine level, and systolic blood pressure. The calculation of a mean or median is an appropriate average. Choices for measures of variability include the range, standard deviation, or standard error.

Variables measured on a ratio scale may be further characterized according to an underlying mathematical model. One such model is the statistically normal or Gaussian distribution. The standard form of this model is the bell-shaped curve shown in Fig. 1. Many familiar statistical analyses require the assumption of this model for their valid application.

Continuous variables can be reduced to a nominal or ordinal scale of measurement. For example, age groups might be constructed as follows: assign to Group 1 those subjects who are less than 18 years of age; to Group 2 those subjects between 18 and 65 years of age; and to Group 3 those subjects over 65 years of age. Age is now measured on an ordinal scale. Age can also be reduced to nominal measurement. One category might be those subjects under 21 years of age, while the other consists of those subjects 21 years of age and older.

If a variable can be measured on a continuous scale, the investigator should record the numerical value. The values can be reclassified subsequently as ordinal or nominal if desired. If the data are recorded initially in categories, the actual values may not be recoverable.

BLINDING OR MASKING

In an unblinded or open study, the researcher and the subject both know which treatment the subject is receiving. Some studies can be done only in this fashion. Although a sham surgical procedure is possible, it is unlikely to be used as a comparison treatment for surgery in humans. Studies that involve changes in exercise and diet are other types of studies conducted on an unblinded basis. Even in an open study, it is appropriate that any laboratory assessments be carried out by technical personnel who are unaware of the subject's treatment.

A single-blind study is one in which the subject does not know which treatment he or she is receiving but the investigator does. A double-blind study is one in which neither the subject nor the care-giver knows which treatment the subject is receiving. (Similar studies involving ophthalmological treatments are usually referred to as "double-masked.") The object of a double-blind study is to remove the investigator's as well as the subject's bias with regard to any study data, particularly if a measurement is subjective.

Carrying out a blinded study requires that the medications be identical in appearance, smell, taste, method of administration, and so forth. A double-blind

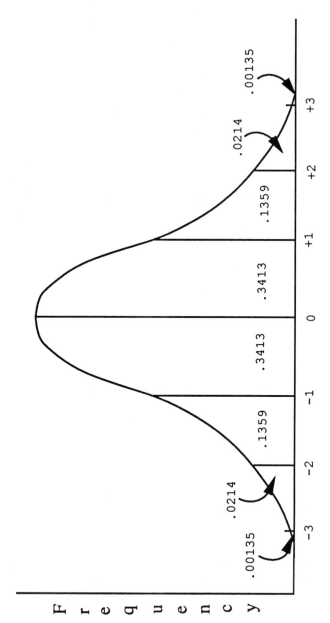

FIG. 1. Statistically normal distribution with mean = 0 and standard deviation = 1.

study is not realistic when one of the treatments has a distinctive side effect or a route of administration different from the other.

A blinded study adds to the complexity of the study administration. For the subjects' health and safety, information about treatment must be readily available through a responsible nonparticipant.

DATA COLLECTION FORMS

Collecting accurate and consistent information about all study subjects is of utmost importance. Data may be accumulated on paper forms, entered directly into a computer using a database package, or transferred directly from one computer to another. For purposes of this discussion, the form may be on paper or on a computer.

It is important to consider carefully the information that must be recorded—demographic information, clinical history, laboratory values, treatment-related information, and so forth. Even items related to the inclusion or exclusion criteria should be included so that the appropriateness of the subjects as study participants can be confirmed later. The investigator should make certain that items which answer the primary and secondary research questions are part of the collected information.

Where possible, the use of check-off categories for variables measured on a nominal or ordinal scale speeds up the data recording process. Although numerical measurements can be categorized in a variety of ways during the analysis phase, it is better to report numerical measurements as actual values rather than categorizing them (e.g., blood pressure is "125/75" instead of "normal"). A number of suggestions for constructing a data collection form are listed in Table 1.

Even if it is expected that only one person will be recording data on the form, for consistency of data interpretation and recording over time it is reasonable to include definitions and criteria for items on the form itself or on a separate instruction form. Normal ranges might be specified so that any out-of-range value is obvious at the time it is recorded. It can be corrected more easily then. Including definitions and normal ranges helps catch errors but does not replace overall quality control of the collected data.

Compiling a "data dictionary" can be extremely helpful. All items of information to be collected are listed with format and possible values [e.g., M or F for male and female, XX.X (0.0 to 15.0) for serum creatinine level, XXX (0 to 275) for systolic or diastolic blood pressure]. In addition, it is useful to include reasonable ranges of values, coding systems, definitions, and other

TABLE 1. CHARACTERISTICS OF GOOD DATA COLLECTION FORMS

- Have clear instructions.
- Include a subject identification and page number on all pages.
- Have a space for date if the same form will be used for several follow-ups.
- Number all items.
- Use lower and upper case text for readability.
- Include a reasonable amount of white space on the form.
- Include data sufficient to attain study goals.
- Make sure questions allow the primary and secondary research questions to be answered.
- Have several simple questions rather than one complex question.
- Where possible, list values to be recorded in the same order as the source document.
- List reasonable range of values for any numerical answers.
- List items for check-off:
    Include "Other" with space for explanation
    Include "Not Applicable" or "Not Done" where appropriate as a response
- Use definitions - even if single person is recording the data.
- Use standardized coding, if possible.
- Include a version number or date of form revision.
- Include a place for the preparer to sign and date.

criteria. Use of the data dictionary over the course of the study will help maintain consistency and accuracy.

When the data collection form and the data dictionary are in final draft form, a "pilot" study should be carried out on a half dozen or so "subjects" to assess the use of the form and the feasibility of the study. Since a pilot study includes relatively few subjects, it is incumbent on the investigator to include some unusual, as well as typical, subjects. Ambiguities and inconsistencies in the use of the form may become apparent.

TESTS OF STATISTICAL HYPOTHESES

Statistical techniques are utilized to provide descriptions of results, to explore associations between two or more measurements, and to make comparisons in such a way that similarity may be established or observed treatment differences may be distinguished from those expected from biological variation.

Much emphasis in the literature has been on the results of statistical hypothesis testing. The current trend is moving toward calculating and reporting confidence intervals, not hypothesis testing. In this section, the philosophy underlying the statistical test of hypotheses will be reviewed, and confidence intervals will be discussed later in this chapter.

The test of statistical hypotheses involves a null and an alternate hypothesis. The null hypothesis is usually one of no difference (e.g., Treatments A and B do not differ in their effects on cholesterol). Paired with the null hypothesis is an alternate hypothesis, which is the complement of the null hypothesis (e.g., Treatments A and B do differ with respect to the effect on cholesterol). The alternate hypothesis stated here is sometimes referred to as two-tailed (or two-sided) because it does not specify which treatment is better. If the researcher has some prior knowledge or a strong belief that one treatment is better than the other, the alternate hypothesis can reflect that information. It would then be referred to as one-sided or one-tailed. The statement of the alternate hypothesis usually reflects the motivation for the research.

Calculations of the test statistic(s) from the data provide the basis for the decision to reject or not to reject the null hypothesis. Referring to Table 2, there are two types of errors that can be made in the decision to reject or not reject the null hypothesis. A Type I, or alpha error, is the error of finding a significant difference when, in reality, there is none. Alpha is the probability of making this error and is usually chosen to be 0.05. Five percent of the time a significant difference will be found when none should.

The second error, a Type II or beta error, is the error of not finding a significant difference when, in reality, there is one. Beta is the probability of making this error. Beta is often chosen to be 0.10 or 0.20. Alpha and beta are related inversely through the sample size; the way to reduce both types of errors is to increase the sample size. Rather than beta, some investigators will specify the power of the statistical test based on the selected sample size. Power is the probability of finding a significant difference when one exists; it can be calculated by subtracting the beta probability from 1.0.

TABLE 2.   ERRORS IN HYPOTHESIS TESTING

Null Hypothesis is:

Decision Based on Data	True	False
Do Not Reject Null Hypothesis	No Error	Type II Error
Reject Null Hypothesis	Type I Error	No Error

Errors and Power

Type I (alpha error) is the error of finding a significant difference when , in reality, there is none.

Type II (beta) error is the error of not finding a significant difference when , in reality, there is one.

Power is the probability of finding a significant difference when one exists.

The investigator often compares treatment groups at the start of a study to support their initial comparability. For the groups to be considered comparable, the investigator would like the results of the comparison of variables that affect the outcome measure to be nonsignificant. (From a practical point of view, a probability or p value of 0.20 or larger supports the comparability of the groups.) For comparison of treatment groups on the major outcome variables, both investigators and journal editors seem to have a strong interest in p values or significance levels of 0.05 or smaller. Since sample size can have a considerable effect on any lack of statistical significance, it is incumbent on the investigator to consider the clinical importance of the results whether they are statistically significant or not.

As noted earlier, a recent trend has been to provide confidence intervals instead of, or in addition to, significance levels. One advantage of a confidence interval is that it provides a set of limits, a reasonable range of values, which is based on the sample size, the observed difference between means (or proportions), and the observed standard deviations. A second advantage is that a 95% confidence interval can be used to infer the results of a two-tailed test of hypothesis at a 5% level of significance.

SAMPLE SIZE SELECTION

There are a variety of approaches to sample size selection. An investigator may chose to do a pilot study, a study of a series of patients larger than any single study in the literature, a study of all available patients with a rare disease, or a study for which the sample sizes were selected on the basis of well-known and accepted statistical standards. In this section I discuss the first three approaches briefly and cover the last in more detail, with references given for further study.

The investigator may wish to treat a very small number of subjects to gain experience or to provide the information for planning a larger study. Such a pilot study with an endpoint measured on a continuous scale might include six to eight subjects in each treatment group. An absolute minimum number is two, the number needed to estimate a standard deviation. If the endpoint is measured on a nominal scale, even a pilot study might need to be much larger. As an example, if a desired endpoint is expected to occur 5% of the time, it would be expected to occur once in 20 subjects. In this case, a pilot study might consist of 60 to 100 subjects per treatment group.

A second approach is to plan a study whose sample size is considerably larger than that of any other study already in the literature. Or, in the case of a rare disease, an investigator might decide to study all of the newly diagnosed subjects with the particular disease entity of interest within a specific time period. Either of these approaches may result in a contribution to knowledge.

The statistical approach to sample size selection requires that the investigator have knowledge of quantitative differences between treatment groups, diagnostic categories, or changes within individuals across doses and times. This might come from the literature or may be obtained from a pilot study or from other local experience. If there is knowledge about the "control" group, then the investigator, in collaboration with a statistician or other more experienced investigators, can select a clinically important difference to detect between control and treated subjects.

Next, the investigator selects acceptable alpha and beta error sizes. The size of alpha error is the probability of finding a significant difference when, in fact, there is none. Usually, the arbitrary choice is 0.05. There may be situations when a 0.10 level is appropriate—in a pilot project, for instance, or in a study where it is impossible to acquire a sample size that would meet more rigorous standards (e.g., in the study of a rare disease).

The choice of a significance level holds for a single statistical comparison. When there are many statistical comparisons to be made, some adjustment must be made in the nominal significance level of an individual comparison (e.g., Bonferroni approach). A professional statistician should be consulted to assess whether this approach is appropriate.

There are times when so many statistical comparisons are planned that a Bonferroni approach may lead to a nominal level of significance of 0.001 or even smaller. In consultation with a statistician, an alternative might be to pick a more stringent significance level, say 0.01, for all comparisons, and state the reason for making this choice.

The beta error is failing to find a significant difference when there is one. Its complement is power, the probability of detecting a significant difference when one exists. It is appropriate to have a statistical test as powerful as possible. A small beta error is desirable. For grant proposals, a beta error of 0.20 (power = 0.80) is generally acceptable.

If an investigator selects a set of study subjects based on an available clinic population or on available care-giving personnel or laboratory resources, the power of the specified sample size can be investigated in advance of the study by consultation with a statistician or reference to *Statistical Tables for the Design of Clinical Trials* (12) or *Statistical Methods for Rates and Proportions* (7). Unless it's a pilot study, the investigator may not wish to proceed if the power of the proposed sample size is less than 50%. An alternative is to find other investigators with similar interests and plan a cooperative study. Many multicenter studies are the result of no single investigator's having sufficient subjects to carry out an important study alone.

Sample size computations can be carried out for the primary outcome measures as well as for the secondary measures. Each computation may yield a different required sample size. The investigator will need to weigh these results in light of priorities as well as the available resources to determine the overall sample size.

In addition to sample size requirements, the investigator needs to consider the willingness of the eligible subjects to agree to participate in the study initially, as well as the attrition of subjects over the course of the study. If 25%

of the entered subjects are expected to be lost over the course of the study, then the investigator should plan on entering 33% more subjects initially.

To determine a starting sample size when the percentage of attrition is known, consider the following:

If N is the total number of subjects required in all groups for a study (based on sample size computations) and X is the percentage of those expected to be lost by attrition, then the total number of subjects M required initially is

$$M = 100 \ N \ / \ (100 - X)$$

If M is not an integer, round up to the nearest multiple of the number of treatment groups.

Two examples of sample size determination are given in this section: the first covers the situation in which there are two groups to be compared and the primary outcome variable is measured on a nominal scale. The second illustrates sample size requirements for the comparison of two groups when the primary response variable is measured on a continuous (or ratio) scale. Equal allocation of subjects to both groups is assumed. When the primary response variable is measured on a nominal scale, the investigator must select alpha and beta and a clinically important difference between the proportions for the control and treatment groups.

Example for Comparing Two Groups When the Response Variable Is Measured on a Nominal Scale

Suppose that the usual 28-day survival rate for a first heart attack in people over 60 years of age is 75% (P1). A new intervention is being considered. The investigators decide that it would be clinically important to detect an improvement to 90% survival (P2) with the new intervention. They plan to study two groups, one treated with the old intervention and a second treated with the new. What sample size *n* in each treatment group is required?

The investigators select alpha = 0.05 and beta = 0.20. Using Table 3 for the appropriate value of AB (= 7.85) and substituting the values for P1 and P2 in the following formula, the required size of each treatment group can be calculated:

$n = AB \times [P1 \times (100 - P1) + P2 \times (100 - P2)] / [(P2 - P1) \times (P2 - P1)]$

$= 7.85 [(75 \times 25) + (90 \times 10)] / [15 \times 15]$

$= 96.8$ or 97 in each treatment group

A total of 194 subjects are needed for both treatment groups.

TABLE 3. VALUES OF AB [*]

		Beta (Type II error)			
		0.05	**0.10**	**0.20**	**0.50**
	0.10	10.82	8.57	6.18	2.71
Alpha (Type I error)	**0.05**	13.00	10.51	7.85	3.84
	0.01	17.81	14.88	11.68	6.63

[*] **THE ALPHA AND BETA FACTOR FOR USE IN DETERMINING SIZE OF EACH   TREATMENT GROUP**

The above formula will give an investigator a good estimate of the required sample size. Fleiss's text provides detailed and more exact tables (7).

When the primary response variable is measured on a continuous scale, the investigator must select alpha, beta, and a clinically important difference between mean values of the response variable expected for the control and treated groups. In addition, the investigator needs an estimate of the standard deviation of the response variable. There are several approaches to obtaining the needed estimate of the standard deviation.

The value of the standard deviation might come from a control or other treated group reported in the literature; it could be estimated from a pilot study; it might also be estimated by taking the range of possible values the measurement can take and dividing by 4. It is useful to make a second sample size computation based on a larger, but still reasonable, standard deviation and to assess whether the additional subjects could be accommodated with the personnel, resources, and time period planned.

It would complicate the sample size determinations if the standard deviations were very different in the control group relative to the treatment group. The approach taken here is that the standard deviations are considered equal for both treatment groups.

Example for Comparing Two Groups When the Response Variable Is Measured on a Continuous Scale

Suppose the investigators were interested in comparing a new serum cholesterol-lowering agent with a standard treatment. With the standard treatment, a decrease of 50 mg/dL was the mean change for a study that appeared in the literature. The standard deviation (SD) of this average change was 15 mg/dL. The investigators believe that lowering serum cholesterol an additional 20 mg/dL would be clinically important. This clinically important difference will be designated as CID. The investigators were satisfied to use alpha = 0.05 as the significance level and selected beta = 0.10.

A minimum sample size for each of two treatment groups can be estimated from the formula given below:

$$n = (AB) [2 \times SD \times SD] / [CID \times CID]$$

$$= 10.51 (2 \times 15 \times 15) / (20 \times 20)$$

$$= 11.8 \text{ or } 12 \text{ in each treatment group.}$$

Thus, at least 12 subjects are required in each group or a total of 24 for both groups.

The text by Machin and Campbell (12) is excellent for determining sample sizes in a variety of clinical trial situations. Computer programs are also available (5).

SUBJECT RETENTION AND COMPLIANCE

When study subjects must be followed on an outpatient basis, their compliance and retention need to be considered in light of the intervention. The investigator may wish to designate a member of the study team (e.g., secretary, social worker, or research nurse) to remind the subject of an upcoming appointment. This can be done via postcard or by telephone or both.

Some investigators find it helpful to distribute an individualized appointment schedule at the start of the study and then have study personnel make contact in advance of the appointment. This may be crucial if follow-up visits are required to occur in a window of time (e.g., a 6-month follow-up must occur 5 to 7 months after the initial intervention).

In addition to compliance with the follow-up visit schedule, it may be important to assess compliance with the treatment. Compliance can be assessed by the subject's self-report. If the study involves medication and it is dispensed by study personnel, the actual amount of medication dispensed can be compared to the expected.

Pill counting is another compliance assessment option, but the investigator must realize that extra pills can be discarded. Additionally, the investigator can schedule laboratory work that would detect a medication in the blood or urine. In a "blinded or masked" study, doing this while maintaining the blind is tricky; in an "open" study, it is less of a problem.

PILOT STUDIES

Once planning the study is completed, it is important that an investigator (new or experienced) carry out a feasibility or pilot study before embarking on the actual study. All of the study methods need to be tested on subjects comparable to those who will be studied under conditions similar to the actual study. This will determine whether the study can be carried out as planned and whether the desired results can be obtained. The results of the pilot study provide a basis for revising study methods.

The data forms should be assessed as discussed earlier in the chapter. If needed, this pilot study can provide information for refining sample size requirements.

METHODS OF STATISTICAL ANALYSIS

Since statistical packages are widely available on computers and statisticians can be consulted at most medical centers, the details of the techniques themselves are not as important as understanding the philosophy and assumptions of statistical techniques.

Statistical methods are utilized to provide summary descriptive information, to explore relationships between two or more variables, and to make comparisons between two or more groups. The new investigator will find useful overviews of statistical methods in publications by the *British Journal of Medicine* (19) and by the Mayo Clinic (14). The *Primer of Biostatistics* (10) and *Biostatistics in Clinical Medicine* (11) are suggested for further development of the new investigator's statistical understanding. *Practical Statistics for Medical Research* (2) is a thorough and medically oriented text, whereas *Biostatistical Analysis* (20) provides a biological, but not necessarily medical, framework with worked examples, extensive tables, and some specialized statistical techniques not ordinarily found in "introductory" texts. Multivariate techniques are covered in an excellent book by Afifi and Clark (1).

The statistical approaches may be characterized as parametric or nonparametric (distribution-free). Parametric statistical tests are ones that have strong and/or extensive assumptions underlying their use. One such strong assumption is that of underlying statistical normality of the target population from which the sample was obtained (Fig. 1). Even when underlying statistical normality is not an appropriate assumption, the population of sample means each based on a sample size of 30 or greater has a distribution that is approximately statistically normal. Thus, parametric techniques can be used to compare means statistically.

When the sample size is small and the assumption of underlying statistical normality is unreasonable, or when the scale of measurement is ordinal or nominal, nonparametric (or distribution-free) techniques are recommended. These tests of hypothesis have fewer and weaker underlying assumptions than their parametric analogs. The assumptions usually involve independence of observations and underlying continuity of the variable under study even though the measurement may be expressed on an ordinal or even nominal basis.

A drawback of nonparametric analysis is that it is less powerful than its parametric counterpart when the assumptions underlying the parametric technique are satisfied. Thus, when data could be analyzed appropriately by parametric methods and nonparametric methods are used instead, the results of the nonparametric analysis will be less significant.

Table 4 lists some common statistical tests for comparing independent or related samples, using parametric or nonparametric techniques for two or more groups. Tables 5A and 5B display, in flow chart fashion, descriptive, relational,

TABLE 4. SOME COMMON STATISTICAL TESTS
FOR THE COMPARISON OF TWO OR MORE GROUPS

	Independent Samples	Related Samples
Parametric	**TWO GROUPS** Student's "t" - independent **THREE OR MORE GROUPS** Analysis of variance followed by multiple comparisons tests such as Student Newman Keuls or Dunnett's Test	**TWO GROUPS** Student's "t" - paired **THREE OR MORE GROUPS** Repeated measures analysis of variance

Nonparametric (Distribution-free)	**TWO GROUPS**
	
	Mann Whitney U Test
	Fisher's Exact Probability
	Chi Square Contingency
	   Table Analysis
	Median Test
	
	THREE OR MORE GROUPS
	
	Kruskal Wallis Analysis of
	   Variance
	Chi Square Contingency
	   Table Analysis
	Median Test
		TWO GROUPS
		
		Sign Test
		Wilcoxon Test
		McNemar Test
		
		THREE OR MORE GROUPS
		
		Friedman Two Way
		Analysis of Variance

TABLE 5A. STATISTICAL TECHNIQUES FOR DESCRIPTION AND CORRELATION

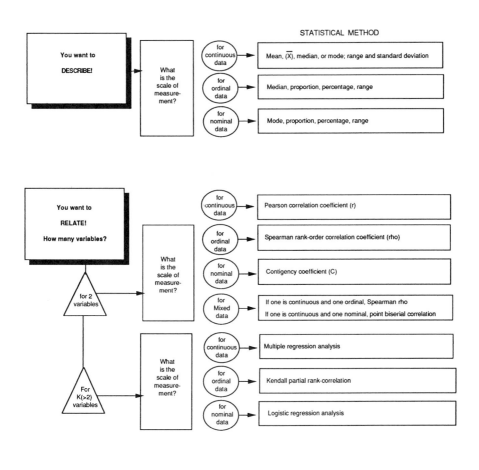

and comparative techniques based on the scale of measurement, the number of groups, and the related or independent nature of the groups (A. C. Elliott, unpublished class notes, 1980). These lists and charts are not intended to be exhaustive. It may be helpful to consult a professional statistician in the planning stages. Appropriate statistical analyses call for preliminary planning to ensure that the research questions can be answered as intended. A text by Rothman (17) provides an excellent introduction on epidemiological concepts, planning studies, and appropriate data analysis.

TABLE 5B. STATISTICAL TECHNIQUES FOR COMPARISON

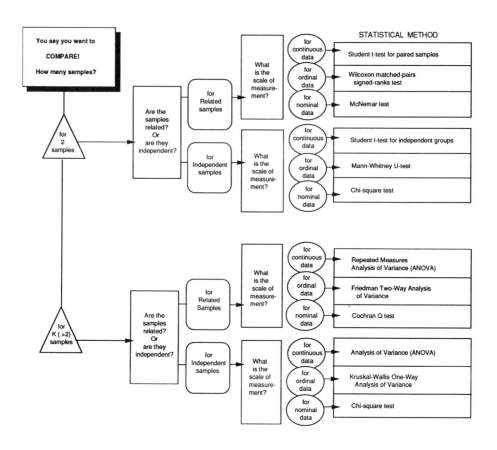

CONFIDENCE INTERVALS

Over the past few years, there has been an increasing trend to report confidence intervals (9) instead of significance levels. The advantage of a confidence interval is that it provides a range of plausible values for an estimate of a difference in treatments (means, proportions, etc.) or of a single estimate (mean, standard deviation, proportion, correlation coefficient, odds ratio, etc.). Quite often, a 95% confidence interval is constructed. This can be related to a two-tailed test of hypothesis at the 5% level of significance (any observed value within the confidence limits would not be significant at the 0.05 level; any value outside the confidence limits would result in a significance level of 0.05 or less).

The statistical interpretation of a 95% confidence interval for a particular value is that if many such intervals are constructed for samples of the same size from the same population, 95% of such intervals will contain the true value of the specified difference somewhere within each set of limits.

A confidence interval is constructed from the estimate of the population value, the standard deviation from the sample, the sample size, and a factor related to the degree of confidence desired. While 95% is a common choice for the degree of confidence, an investigator may wish to construct a 90% or a 99% confidence level instead of or in addition. The interval is narrower when the degree of confidence is relaxed (say 90% or less) and is wider as the degree of confidence is increased.

Four examples are presented to illustrate the computations. The confidence limits for the proportion examples are valid when the product of the sample size, the observed proportion, and 1.0 minus the observed proportion is at least 5. Check the validity before computing by calculating $N \times P \times (1 - P)$ and making sure it has a value of 5 or larger.

Example of a 95% Confidence Interval for a Single Proportion

If a researcher wants to estimate what proportion of mothers breast feed their babies for at least the first 6 weeks of life, he or she might survey 200 (N1) mothers who bring their babies to well baby clinic during a particular 2-week period. Suppose it is found that 32% (P1 = 0.32) of the mothers respond affirmatively. A similar survey done during another 2-week period is likely to yield a different result. Checking for validity, $N1 \times P1 \times (1 - P1)$ is computed and found to be 43.52; a valid 95% confidence interval can be calculated. A reasonable range of values for the proportion of breast-feeding mothers in the target population represented by that week's sample can be calculated from the following:

Lower Limit:

$$P1 - 1.96 \times \sqrt{\frac{P1 \times (1-P1)}{N1}}$$

Upper Limit:

$$P1 + 1.96 \times \sqrt{\frac{P1 \times (1-P1)}{N1}}$$

The value "1.96" is a constant appropriate for a 95% confidence interval. Different degrees of confidence require other values (90% confidence: 1.645; 99% confidence: 2.282).

Thus, the lower 95% confidence limit is

$$= 0.32 - 1.96 \times \sqrt{\frac{0.32 \times 0.68}{200}}$$
$$= 0.32 - 0.065$$
$$= 0.255$$

And the upper limit is

$$= 0.32 + 0.065$$
$$= 0.385$$

Based on this sample of 200 mothers, the true percentage of breast-feeding mothers in the target population could be as small as 25.5% or as high as 38.5%. This statement is made with 95% confidence.

Example of a 95% Confidence Interval for the Difference Between Two Proportions

An investigator is interested in comparing povidone-iodine (Betadine®) to sterile saline in cleansing lacerations for patients who come to the emergency room of a large city hospital. The outcome measure is the presence of an infection in the laceration at a 3- to 7-day follow-up visit. Since it is expected that only 50% of the patients will return for the follow-up visit, a total of 2,000 subjects are randomized equally to the two methods using a sealed envelope method. (When an eligible patient agrees to participate in the research study, the next opaque envelope is opened and the cleansing agent listed inside is utilized.)

About 2% to 5% of the subjects whose lacerations are cleansed with povidone-iodine are expected to have infections at follow-up. It is hypothesized that sterile saline will have similar results. At the completion of the study, 26 of 550 ($P1 = 0.047$; $N1 = 550$) subjects who received sterile saline are found to have an infection, and 20 of the 475 ($P2 = 0.042$; $N2 = 475$) subjects whose lacerations were cleansed with povidone-iodine had infections. The true difference between infection rates is estimated by the following 95% confidence limits:

Lower Limit:

$$P1 - P2 - 1.96 \times \sqrt{\frac{P1 \times (1-P1)}{N1} + \frac{P2 \times (1-P2)}{N2}}$$

Upper Limit:

$$P1 - P2 + 1.96 \times \sqrt{\frac{P1 \times (1-P1)}{N1} + \frac{P2 \times (1-P2)}{N2}}$$

Thus, the lower limit is

$$= 0.047 - 0.042 - 1.96 \times$$

$$\sqrt{\frac{0.047 \times 0.953}{550} + \frac{0.042 \times 0.958}{475}}$$

$$= 0.005 - 1.96 \times 0.013$$
$$= 0.005 - 0.025$$
$$= -0.020$$

And the upper limit is

$$= 0.005 + 0.025$$
$$= 0.030$$

Based on this sample of 1,025 subjects, the true difference in the target population (subjects who come to this large city hospital for treatment of lacerations) could be as much as 2.0% more infections with cleansing with povidone-iodine or 3.0% fewer infections with povidone-iodine. This statement is made with 95% confidence. Since the value "0.0" is included within the confidence limits, a test of the null hypothesis comparing these two treatments would not have been rejected at the 0.05 level of significance (i.e., the difference in the outcomes with the two agents was not statistically significant).

Example of 95% Confidence Interval for a Mean

A researcher treating subjects for hypertriglyceridemia decides to study a new treatment designed to reduce triglycerides. Subjects taking part in the study have had triglyceride levels consistently above 300 mg/dL for 6 months despite having been counseled to make dietary changes. Twenty-five (N) subjects agree to take part in the study, and at their follow-up visit, 1 month after starting treatment, the average reduction is 155 mg/dL (MEAN DIF) with a standard deviation of 60 mg/dL (SD).

Based on the results for these subjects, what is a reasonable range of reduction in triglyceride values in a target population of similar subjects? The 95% confidence limits are calculated as follows.

Upper Limit:

$$Mean\ Dif - \frac{t \times SD}{\sqrt{N}}$$

Lower Limit:

$$Mean\ Dif + \frac{t \times SD}{\sqrt{N}}$$

[t (Student's t) is a factor related to the sample size; values of Student's t for determining 95% confidence limits are included in Table 6; appropriate values of Student's t *depend on a constant called* degrees of freedom *(DF); in this situation DF = N - 1 = 24.]*

Thus, the lower limit is

$$= 155 - \frac{2.064 \times 60}{\sqrt{25}}$$

$$= 155 - 25$$
$$= 130$$

And the upper limit is

$$= 155 + 25$$
$$= 130$$

Based on this sample of 25 subjects, the reduction in triglyceride level in the target population could be as low as 130 mg/dL or as high as 180 mg/dL with 95% confidence in making this statement. This reduction was "statistically significant at the 0.05 level," since a value of zero (no reduction) was outside the 95% confidence limits.

TABLE 6. VALUES OF "t" FOR CALCULATING 95%
CONFIDENCE LIMIT

DF	t	DF	t
1	12.706	21	2.080
2	4.303	22	2.074
3	3.182	23	2.069
4	2.776	24	2.064
5	2.571	25	2.060
6	2.447	26	2.056
7	2.365	27	2.052
8	2.306	28	2.048
9	2.262	29	2.045
10	2.228	30	2.042
11	2.201	40	2.021
12	2.179	50	2.009
13	2.160	60	2.000
14	2.145	70	1.994
15	2.131	80	1.990
16	2.120	90	1.987
17	2.110	100	1.984
18	2.101	>100	1.960
19	2.093		
20	2.086		

Example of a 95% Confidence Interval for the Difference Between Two Independent Means

An investigator is interested in comparing two different approaches to weight loss for subjects who are more than 25% over their recommended weight for their sex, height, and age. The 100 available subjects are stratified by sex and randomized equally into two groups within each stratum. Subjects are instructed in the weight loss program to which they were assigned and are instructed to maintain their current physical activity level.

Subjects weigh in weekly and the success of the weight loss program is judged by the average weight loss at the end of 2 months. The groups had similar average weights at the start of the study period.

The results were that the members of Group 1 (N1 = 43) lost an average of 16 pounds (MEAN1) with a standard deviation of 4.5 pounds (SD1); the members of Group 2 (N2 = 42) lost an average of 10 pounds (MEAN2) with a standard deviation of 3.2 pounds (SD2).

The 95% confidence limits for the mean weight loss between the two approaches is calculated as follows.

Lower Limit:

$$MEAN1\text{-}MEAN2 - t \times SP \times \sqrt{\frac{1}{N1} + \frac{1}{N2}}$$

Upper Limit:

$$MEAN1\text{-}MEAN2 + t \times SP \times \sqrt{\frac{1}{N1} + \frac{1}{N2}}$$

where

$$SP = \sqrt{\frac{(N1\text{-}1) \times SD1^2 + (N2\text{-}1) \times SD2^2}{N1 + N2 - 2}}$$

and Student's t is based on DF = N1 + N2 - 2. First SP is calculated.

$$SP = \sqrt{\frac{42 \times 45^2 + 41 \times 3.2^2}{43 + 42 - 2}}$$

$$= \sqrt{\frac{850.50 + 419.84}{83}}$$

$$= \sqrt{15.305}$$

$$= 3.912$$

Then, the 95% confidence limits are calculated.

Lower Limit:

$$= 16\text{-}10\text{-}1.99 \times 3.912 \times \sqrt{\frac{1}{43} + \frac{1}{42}}$$

$$= 6\text{-}1.99 \times 3.912 \times 0.217$$
$$= 6\text{-}1.7$$
$$= 4.3$$

Upper Limit:

$$= 6+1.7$$
$$= 7.7$$

Based on these samples the difference for the true weight loss between the two programs could be as little as 4.3 pounds or as much as 7.7 pounds. This statement is made with 95% confidence. The difference between the two approaches to weight loss is significant at the 0.05 level, since the value zero (no difference between programs) is outside the confidence limits.

SITE VISITS

Table 7 outlines topics related to statistical issues about which an investigator should be knowledgeable in planning a study, in discussing at a site visit, and in writing the manuscript for publication. This table was adapted from a list of questions I received shortly before an NIH site visit for a program-project grant.

PUBLICATION

A well-planned and executed clinical study is a contribution to the literature and to science. In Chapter 10, Dr. Grundy provides excellent advice about overall manuscript preparation. The emphasis in this chapter is experimental design and statistical issues. It behooves the investigator to convey the information that went into the design and statistical analysis of the study and its results along with the methodology supporting the clinical design and execution. Reviewers of the manuscript, including experienced researchers as well as statisticians, look for the following elements.

Descriptions of the target population, as well as the sample, should be included along with eligibility/exclusion criteria. The design of the experiment

TABLE 7. ISSUES TO BE ADDRESSED BY PRESENTERS

OF RESEARCH PROTOCOLS

- Hypothesis to be tested.

- Specific research questions asked.

- How will the proposed methods help answer each of the questions.

- Definitions of disease category, improvement, failure, relapse, response, resistance to treatment, etc.

- What are the methods designed to insure the homogeneity of the sample population (e.g. age, sex, previous clinical history, previous treatment history, further therapy, clinical category).

- Number of subjects in each category expected to be contributed by each participating institution.

- Possible pitfalls of the selection process.

- Standardization of the treatment or management intervention.

- Expected duration of the study.

- Estimation of quantitative differences among treatment groups or clinical categories.

- Needed sample sizes based on the above estimates.

- End points.

- Method(s) of statistical analysis.

- New knowledge expected from this study (be specific).

should be described in sufficient detail that it could be repeated if any investigator desired to do so. The method of randomization should be described briefly but convincingly.

It is useful to include a statistical methods section, but this is not sufficient by itself; the method should also be named where a specific result is given in the text or tables. References for the statistical methods (preferably textbooks rather than articles in which methods were used) should be provided for any method that is not common. No references would be expected for Student's t test, chi-square contingency analysis, or Pearson correlation coefficient, but more unfamiliar techniques such as logistic stepwise regression or Kaplan-Meier survival analysis should be referenced. Computer programs, if utilized, should be referenced as well. If one-tailed tests were used, provide a brief justification in the text.

Few journals have space to include all of the basic study data, but summary statistics (means, standard deviations, ranges of values, sample sizes, etc.) that could be utilized by a reader or reviewer to verify reported results and probability values should be provided.

Descriptors should be included for the entire set of data as well as any major subset on which important conclusions are based. In addition to means and standard deviations, observed ranges of values can provide insight to a reader. Tables and graphs should be labeled and clear. It may be helpful to have a collaborating statistician look over the manuscript before submission; this could save revisions later.

Two excellent articles provide detailed guidelines for the necessary elements related to experimental design and statistical analysis to be included in a publication of study results (3,4). Some investigators have published guidelines for judging the published results of clinical trials (6,16). Such guidelines can also be used as a checklist for the new investigator before submitting a manuscript.

CONCLUSION

Statistical principles influence the planning of a clinical study, its execution, and the interpretation of the results. This chapter focused on those principles and provided references for the new investigator's further development.

REFERENCES

1. Afifi, A.A. and Clark, V. (1990): *Computer-aided Multivariate Analysis.* 2nd ed. Van Nostrand Reinhold Company, New York.
2. Altman, D.G. (1991): *Practical Statistics for Medical Research.* Chapman and Hall, New York.
3. Altman, D.G., Gore, S.M., Gardner, M.J., and Pocock, S.J. (1983): Statistical guidelines for contributors to medical journals. *Br. Med. J.* 286:1489–1493.
4. Bailar, J.C., III and Mosteller, F. (1988): Guidelines for statistical reporting in articles for medical journals. *Ann. Intern. Med.* 108:266–273.
5. Borenstein, M. and Cohen, J. (1989): *Statistical Power Analysis.* Release 1.00. Lawrence Erlbaum Associates, Hillsdale, NJ.

6. Chalmers, T.C., Smith, H., Jr., Blackburn, B., Silverman, B., Schroeder, B., Reitman, D., and Ambroz, A. (1981): A method for assessing the quality of a randomized control trial. *Controlled Clin. Trials* 1:31–49.
7. Fleiss, J.L. (1981): *Statistical Methods for Rates and Proportions.* 2nd ed. John Wiley & Sons, New York.
8. Friedman, L.M., Furberg, C.D., and DeMets, D.L. (1981): *Fundamentals of Clinical Trials.* John Wright PSG, Boston.
9. Gardner, M.J. and Altman, D.G. (1986): Confidence intervals rather than P values: estimation rather than hypothesis testing. *Br. Med. J.* 292:746–750.
10. Glantz, S.A. (1992): *Primer of Biostatistics.* 3rd ed. McGraw-Hill, New York.
11. Ingelfinger, J.A., Mosteller, F., Thibodeau, L.A., and Ware, J.H. (1987): *Biostatistics in Clinical Medicine.* 2nd ed. Macmillan Publishing Company, New York.
12. Machin, D. and Campbell, M.J. (1987): *Statistical Tables for the Design of Clinical Trials.* Blackwell Scientific Publications, Boston.
13. Meinert, C.L. (1986): *Clinical Trials: Design, Conduct, and Analysis.* Oxford University Press, New York.
14. O'Brien, P.C. and Shampo, M.A. (1981): *Statistics for Clinicians.* Mayo Foundation, Rochester, MN.
15. Pocock, S.J. (1983): *Clinical Trials: A Practical Approach.* John Wiley & Sons, New York.
16. Reisch, J.S., Tyson, J.E., and Mize, S.G. (1989): Aid to the evaluation of therapeutic studies. *Pediatrics* 84:815–827.
17. Rothman, K.J. (1986): *Modern Epidemiology.* Little, Brown and Company, Boston.
18. Spilker, B. (1991): *Guide to Clinical Trials.* Raven Press, New York.
19. Swinscow, T.D.V. (1980): *Statistics at Square One.* 7th ed. *British Medical Journal,* London.
20. Zar, J.H. (1984): *Biostatistical Analysis.* 2nd ed. Prentice-Hall, Englewood Cliffs, NJ.

7

General Laboratory Techniques in Clinical Research

Joseph E. Zerwekh, Ph.D.

*Center for Mineral Metabolism and Clinical Research, University of Texas
Southwestern Medical Center at Dallas, Dallas, Texas 75235-8885*

Successful conduction of clinical research requires the application of specific laboratory techniques. A consideration of all the available techniques and methods that are currently available to the clinical researcher is beyond the scope of this presentation. Obviously, investigators will require their own armamentariums of laboratory methods that are particularly suited to their individual areas of investigation. Most of these methods represent general techniques rather than molecular biological approaches. Thus, in this chapter I will present general laboratory procedures that are currently available to the clinical investigator and discuss their advantages and disadvantages. It is hoped that this consideration will aid the novice clinical investigator in choosing the laboratory techniques that can provide sensitive, accurate, economical, and reproducible measurements in the execution of clinical research.

SPECIMEN COLLECTION AND HANDLING

Clinical research can be categorized as basic clinical research, patient-oriented research, clinical trials, epidemiology, and clinical observation. Despite the many faces of clinical research, the unifying factor is that clinical research involves human subjects. Thus, most, if not all, laboratory techniques will utilize specimens from human subjects.

The accuracy, sensitivity, and reproducibility of laboratory analysis depend on the condition of the specimen. For this reason reliable laboratory determinations in clinical research start with good specimen collection and preservation. This tenet holds true for all clinical specimens, including urine, stool, saliva, blood, and tissue, to name but a few.

The rate of production and breakdown of substances in the body and their concentrations in the body fluids are influenced by a multitude of factors, such as intake of meals, posture, and time of day. The concentrations of substances in the specimens are influenced by various factors including the gauge of needles used for venipuncture, whether open or vacuum blood collection tubes are utilized, and the additives contained in the specimen collection vessels. Following its collection, the specimen may be treated in various ways (e.g., separation of clot from plasma, centrifugation, freezing, thawing, and division of the specimen into smaller samples for subsequent analysis). The factors influencing the results of a laboratory assay between the procurement of the specimen and analysis proper are called *preanalytical* factors.

It is convenient to divide the preanalytical factors into *in vivo* or biological factors and *in vitro* factors. The *in vivo* factors act in the subject prior to or during specimen collection and can cause variation in the composition of body fluids and tissues. A partial listing of some of these biological factors is presented in Table 1. These factors may be divided into two groups, those that can and those that cannot be "influenced." To the latter belong sex, age, race, and similar factors. These factors are commonly used to partition the reference individuals into groups. Important factors that one can influence are (a) meals and prolonged fasting; (b) the intake of pharmacologically active substances including drugs, hormones, ethanol, caffeine, and tobacco; (c) hemodynamic factors including posture; and (d) cell and tissue damage induced by physical work, muscle massage, and venipuncture. To reduce the possible adverse effects of these controllable factors on the study outcome, it is best to obtain specimens under a controlled environment such as that found at the general clinical research center. In addition, use of the general clinical research center can also greatly reduce the *in vitro* or methodological variation in specimen handling. Specimen procurement and handling are identical, not only from subject to subject but also from specimen to specimen in the same subject.

Table 1. *Factors causing biological variation*

Age	Pharmacologically active agents
Activity	Physical fitness
Altitude	Posture
Blood type	Profession
Body mass and surface	Puberty, menstruation, pregnancy,
Chronobiological rhythms	menopause
Diet (type, amount)	Relation to meals
Disease	Sex
Environment (humidity, temperature)	Socioeconomic class
Ethnic group and race	Specimen collection (site, technique)
Exercise	Stress
Exposure to toxic agents, radiation, etc.	Trauma
Genetic factors	

Table 2 presents a checklist for specimen handling that can be used as an aid in reducing methodological variation. A more detailed narrative as well as specific recommendations can be found in recent publications (10,11).

In general, the type of analyses performed on samples generated from clinical research studies will require one or more of four approaches. They are represented by (a) biochemical or pharmacological techniques, (b) histological techniques, (c) cell culture systems, and (d) molecular (DNA) techniques. A detailed consideration of molecular biological techniques in clinical research will not be discussed here. A consideration of the three remaining general laboratory approaches will be presented.

TABLE 2. *Checklist for specimen handling*

Transport	Storage
—Container, preservatives	—Container
—Temperature	—Preservative, if any
—Duration	—Temperature
Clotting	Preparation for analysis
—Time	—Thawing
—Temperature	—Mixing
—Promoting agent	—Enzymatic digestion
Separation of plasma and serum	
—Centrifugation force and time	
—Temperature	

BIOCHEMICAL (PHARMACOLOGICAL) ANALYSIS

Assay Choice and Development

Biochemical analyses are, by far, the most popular general type of assay. The choice of a particular type of biochemical or pharmacological assay system will be initially dictated by the type of analyte being measured. These analytes fall into two categories, common and specific analytes. Common analytes are usually present in sufficient quantity in the specimen for colorimetric or automated methods to provide the necessary sensitivity and specificity. Many of these assays are performed by reference laboratories and offer an economical alternative to the establishment of a bench procedure in the investigator's own laboratory. Another option may be to enlist the services of the general clinical research center core laboratory, where many of the assays for the common analytes may be routinely performed.

On the other hand, specific analytes are usually present in small quantities (e.g., hormones, growth factors, drugs) and may require the use of more specialized analytical methods. Again, the clinical investigator may wish to utilize the services of an outside laboratory to perform these determinations if deemed cost-effective. If a large number of determinations is anticipated, it may be more practical to purchase a commercial kit for the specific analyte. These kit procedures generally can accommodate 25 to 40 specimens. However, a majority of these commercially available kit assays require familiarity with isotope handling and monitoring. Finally, if none of the above options is applicable, then the investigator must consider the development of the necessary assay(s).

Before an assay can be developed and instituted in an investigator's laboratory, three questions should be asked: (a) Can the analyte(s) in question be isolated and measured by standard biochemical techniques such as gel chromatography, high-pressure liquid chromatography (HPLC), colorimetric reactions, and enzymatic reactions? (b) Is the method reproducible, accurate, sensitive, time-saving, and cost-effective? (c) Is antibody (polyclonal or monoclonal) to the analyte available? If not, can the analyte be used as an antigen for the generation of antisera and/or labeled with an appropriate indicator for the development of an immunoassay? The answers to these questions may limit the investigator to a specific type of assay, or the investigator may be faced with the option of developing a totally new biochemical assay procedure. In general, three types of assay systems can be explored as possible methods—the bioassay, chemical assay, and immunoassay.

Bioassay

Bioassay quantitatively determines an analyte by measuring its specific bioactivity in a target system and comparing the response to that produced by known concentrations of the analyte. An example of bioassay is the "line test," wherein the antirachitic activity of various vitamin D metabolites can be quantitatively determined. It is performed by dosing rachitic rats with the isolated vitamin D analog (e.g., from serum) along with standard amounts of the vitamin D metabolite in question. After several days the width of the mineralization front (line) is measured in the metaphyseal area of a long bone. The width of the line is directly proportional to the concentration of vitamin D administered. Cells in culture can also be used as the target system to quantitatively determine the biological response to various analytes. Although bioassays can provide detection at extremely low levels for some analytes, they are generally time-consuming and require the isolation and partial purification of the analyte from the specimen.

Chemical Assay

Chemical assays take advantage of a specific chemical (biochemical) reaction or physical property of the analyte. The success of this type of assay is usually dependent on a particular structural or biochemical property of the analyte. Like the bioassay, the observed response is compared to that produced by standard concentrations of the analyte. The colorimetric determination of protein is a classic example of a chemical reaction. Quantitative determination of an analyte's enzymatic properties would represent a biochemical assay. High-pressure liquid chromatographic quantitative determination of certain drugs would represent a widely used physical technique. Many of these chemical assays can provide extremely low levels of detection but sometimes require prior isolation and partial purification of the analyte from its specimen. These assays tend to be less time-consuming than bioassays but may necessitate the procurement of specialized and sometimes expensive equipment.

Immunoassay

Quantitative analytical methods with antibodies or antigens as primary reagents are now integral to many clinical, pharmaceutical, and basic scientific investigations. For numerous clinically important analytes that are proteins or peptides (including many hormones, lipoproteins, oncoproteins, pathogenic antigens, and specific antibodies), there are, as yet, no viable alternatives. Even where an analyte can feasibly be determined by chromatographic, colorimetric, or other standard procedures, quantitative immunological methods (i.e., immunoassays) are often used because of their speed, simplicity, and relatively low cost. This trend has been greatly encouraged by the availability of convenient, reliable commercial kits.

Most immunoassays can readily be shown to be either "limited reagent" (i.e., competitive, antigen excess) methods because they make use of limited amounts of antibody or "reagent excess" (i.e., noncompetitive antibody excess) methods in which, as in most classic methods of chemical analysis, the primary reagents are in excess. However, an increasing number of variations are to be found in clinical laboratories and a much greater number are encountered in

TABLE 3. *Classification of immunoassays:heterogeneous vs. homogeneous*

Classification	Type of immunoassay	Relative antigen-antibody concentration
Heterogeneous immunoassay		
—Competitive saturation immunoassay	RIA (Yalow and Berson) Solid phase RIA Competitive EIA	Antigen excess
—Immunometric assay	Immunoradiometric assay (IRMA-Miles and Hale) Immunoenzymometric	Antibody excess
—Sandwich immunoassay	Two-site immunoradiometric assay (two-site IRMA) Sandwich EIA	Antibody excess
Homogeneous immunoassay		
	Fluorescence excitation transfer assay	Antibody excess
	Fluorescence polarization immunoassay	Antigen excess

research reports and papers. The classification, presented in Table 3, divides immunoassays into two broad groups, heterogeneous and homogeneous immunoassays. This terminology was proposed to distinguish between immunoassays that required separation of the bound and free fraction to obtain a result (i.e., heterogeneous) and immunoassays in which separation was not required (i.e., homogeneous). The different types of heterogeneous immunoassays are defined by general terms irrespective of the indicator used to signal the reaction (i.e., radioactivity, enzymic activity, or fluorescence). As a guide, the names of some of the immunoassays which fit into these categories are also presented. The names of homogeneous assays are listed separately because of their restricted use and diverse design.

The rationale for this classification is based on the difference in the binding strength of an antibody-combining site (affinity) and the entire molecule (activity) for antigen. Generally speaking, the activity of antibody can be 1,000 to 10,000 times stronger than the affinity of the combining site of the same

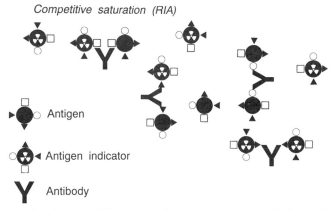

FIG.1. Schematic of competitive saturation immunoassay depicting the relative concentrations of antigen (excess) and antibody during the initial incubation of antigen and antibody.

antibody for an antigenic determinant. This difference, in part, reflects the ability of both antibody-combining sites of IgG to bind antigen. Dissociation of a determinant from one antibody-combining site may not mean dissociation of the antibody from the antigen, since the other combining site may still be bound to the antigen. In contrast, affinity measurements are made in the presence of excess antigen so that multivalent interactions of antibody with antigen are minimized, which, in turn, means that the antigen-antibody binding represents the energy of interaction between a combining site and an antigenic determinant. A hypothetical illustration of this concept is presented in Figs. 1 and 2, which

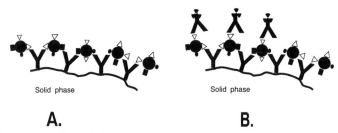

A.   **B.**

FIG. 2. Schematic of sandwich immunoassay demonstrating the antibody (excess) with bound antigen during initial incubation conditions (**A**) and the addition of a second antibody carrying the radioactive indicator (**B**). Symbols are identical to those for Figure 1.

contrast extremes in design of immunoassay systems that rely on the affinity (e.g., a conventional radioimmunoassay) or activity (e.g., a sandwich immunoassay) of the antibody molecule to bind to a protein antigen.

Figure 1 illustrates the situation found in the conventional radioimmunoassay (RIA) initially described by Yalow and Berson (14), which uses limiting concentrations of antibody and an excess concentration of antigen. These assays are usually set up so that 50% of the radiolabeled antigen is bound by the antibody. Addition of increasing amounts of cold antigen to the assay displaces the radiolabeled antigen from the antibody, which, in turn, can be quantitatively determined to show the concentration of antigen in an unknown. Limiting the antibody concentration in this assay means that each antibody-combining site will be bound to a separate antigen molecule, which minimizes the possibility of multiple interactions of a number of antibodies with an antigen molecule. Dissociation of an antigenic determinant from an antibody-combining site results in the site being unoccupied by antigen until another antigenic determinant of the antigen presents itself in the correct orientation to bind to the site again. The degree of cross-reactivity seen in this immunoassay is directly proportional to the difference in the affinity of the antibody for the homologous and heterologous antigenic determinant.

Figure 2 illustrates the converse situation found in a sandwich immunoassay. These assays are set up in antibody excess, with antibody bound to the solid phase "extracting" the antigen out of solution. The solid phase is washed to remove unbound protein, with the bound antigen detected by the addition of antibody containing an indicator molecule (e.g., radioisotope, enzyme, or fluorescent molecule). The concentration of antigen detected in this assay is directly proportional to the amount of antibody indicator bound to the solid phase. The use of excess antibody in the solid phase extraction and at the antibody indicator stage favors the development of multiple interactions of many antibodies with one antigen molecule. During the initial incubation of the assay, antigens will associate first and then dissociate from the antibody on the solid phase until multiple interactions with the antibody have occurred to hold the antigen firmly to the solid phase. This "cross-linking" leads to antigen-antibody bonds that are stronger than the "univalent bonds" that occur in conventional RIAs. If an antigenic determinant of an antigen dissociates from one antibody-combining site, there are always others to hold the antigen to the solid phase. Thus, dissociation of the antigen is difficult, and it is probable that a dissociated determinant will reoccupy the same combining site. This design leads to immunoassays that are theoretically more sensitive than RIA. However, sandwich assays will show a higher degree of cross-reactivity than RIA for these same reasons. Multiple interactions of many antibodies with an inappropriate antigen that contains heterologous antigenic determinants could bind to the solid phase absorbent and give a false-positive result. Thus, antigenic discrimination by these assays could be minimal.

Immunoassay Development

Antibody Development

Before an investigator can decide which type of immunoassay system might best serve his or her research needs, a consideration of antibody development must be made. If a commercially available antibody is to be used, the investigator must ascertain that the antibody has the appropriate specificity for the antigen in question. If it is found to be suitable, the investigator should ensure that there is a sufficient amount of the material available to perform the anticipated number of assays. If no antibody is available and production is required, the question of whether to develop polyclonal or monoclonal antibodies must be considered.

Monoclonal Antibodies

The discovery and development of monoclonal antibodies, as by Kohler and Milstein (4), has extended the horizon of scientific investigation in a diverse number of disciplines. The ability to generate the same antibody in copious amounts and for an indefinite period led to the standardization and refinement of immunoassay in clinical research.

The monoclonal antibody technique involves the random fusion of lymphoid cells from an immunized mouse with a mouse plasmacytoma cell line adapted to grow in cell culture. After fusion, the cells are divided into portions and cultured separately. Selective growth of the lymphoid-plasmacytoma hybrid cell (i.e., hybridoma) is accomplished by correction of a metabolic defect in the plasmacytoma cell line by genetic information contributed by the lymphoid cell. Plasmacytoma cells fail to grow in selective tissue culture media, whereas the lymphoid cells die because of their inability to adapt to cell culture.

Culture supernatant fluids from the hybridomas must be assayed for the production of the appropriate antibody because some hybridomas will not produce antibody while others will secrete an inappropriate antibody. These "screening immunoassays" must be performed when growth of the hybridoma appears so that overgrowth of the culture by nonsecreting hybridomas can be minimized. Hybridomas producing an acceptable antibody are then isolated by using techniques analogous to those used for bacteria. These "cloning steps" are usually performed twice to assure the monoclonality of the cell population. A monoclonal hybridoma cell line can be frozen in liquid nitrogen and stored indefinitely. These cells will produce up to 100 µg of antibody per mL of culture fluid when grown *in vitro* or up to 10 mg of antibody per mL of ascitic fluid when grown *in vivo* in mice.

From a practical standpoint, the production of monoclonal antibodies is very expensive in terms of cost of personnel and material to maintain the cell cultures and the time it takes to achieve a product. Second, the success of producing the appropriate monoclonal antibody for an immunoassay is not always guaranteed. The success of the technique is dependent upon the number of B cells producing antibody of the appropriate affinity to the immunogen. High-affinity antibodies comprise 1% to 3% of the antibodies in an antiserum. If it is assumed that the same proportion of cells secrete these antibodies, the isolation of a hybridoma producing high-affinity antibody would be difficult.

These considerations also stress the importance of the proper choice of which immunoassay is used in screening the hybridoma before cloning steps are initiated. The immunoassays used should be identical or similar in principle to the immunoassay that is being developed. Monoclonal antibodies may not react identically in all types of immunoassays. Moreover, the antibody may be difficult to purify from ascitic fluid or could be inactivated by procedures used to covalently attach indicator molecules. All of these aspects must be investigated as early as possible in the procedure to minimize the amount of work invested on an unsuitable monoclonal antibody. Thus, it is not surprising that the success rate for generating appropriate monoclonal antibodies for difficult antigens has been found to be one to three per year per worker in a laboratory that is producing monoclonal antibodies full time.

Polyclonal Antibodies

For illustrative purposes, polyclonal and monoclonal antibodies can be considered mirror images of each other. The advantages and limitations of each antibody population are presented in Table 4.

The cost and time invested in preparation of polyclonal antibodies are minimal by comparison to monoclonal antibodies. A large number of animals can be immunized and periodically boosted with antigen, and the antisera can be tested for the appearance of the appropriate population of antibody. Large volumes of antisera are not required to perform thousands of RIAs if the antibody is of the appropriate affinity. Thus, if the antigen is immunogenic, it is probable that an antisera can be obtained for an immunoassay.

The major theoretic limitation of monoclonal antibodies is that they are less selective than polyclonal antibodies because one antibody defines antigen. Furthermore, if a monoclonal antibody is developed for an immunoassay and a cross-reactivity is found which compromises the selectivity of the assay, the monoclonal antibody is useless. Adsorption of the monoclonal antibody with the cross-reacting antigen is ineffective, since each antibody in the population will react with antigen to the same degree. In contrast, cross-reactive antibodies in an antiserum (polyclonal) can be removed by adsorption of antibody with cross-

TABLE 4. *Comparison of monoclonal and polyclonal antibodies*

Monoclonal antibodies	Polyclonal antibodies
Limitations	*Advantages*
—Expensive in cost and time	—Inexpensive in cost and time
—Questionable success of product	—Reliable success of product
—Less selective: one antibody defines antigen	—More selective: diverse number of antibodies define antigen
—Cross-reactivity cannot be removed	—Cross-reactivity removed by adsorption
—Antibody reacts with one facet of an antigenic determinant	—Antibodies react with all facets of antigenic determinant
—Each has unique biochemical characteristics	—Common biochemical characteristics
Advantages	*Limitations*
—Stable antibody product	—Dynamic antibody production in each antisera
—Source of antibody immortal	—Population of antibody short-lived
—Antibody produced in large amounts	—Antibody present in limited amounts
—Homogeneous affinity	—Heterogeneous affinity
—Can artificially manipulate antibody	—Cannot manipulate antibody
—Crude immunogen for immunization	—Highly purified antigen for immunization
—Excellent reagent for antigen purification	—Poor reagent for antigen purification

reacting antigen without affecting other antibodies that react with the homologous antigen.

The advantages of obtaining the appropriate monoclonal antibody for immunoassay can surpass their limitations, discussed above. The advantages they have over polyclonal antibodies will not be considered, since many of these points are obvious and are more thoroughly discussed in specific publications (2,5,8,12).

COMPARISON OF INDICATORS

Radioisotopes, fluorophores, or enzymes have been the indicators used primarily to prepare tracers for the immunoassays to be described below. Some of the indicators are better suited for certain types of immunoassays than others. The advantages and limitations of the three major indicators will be briefly reviewed before analyzing the different types of immunoassays (Table 5).

Radioisotopes

The limitations of radioisotopes are inherent and unique to this type of indicator. *Decay catastrophe* refers to the damage that occurs to the tracer when the radioactive atom decays. There may then be molecular damage, which may compromise the immunoreactivity of the tracer. This damage can be minimized by incorporating an average of one radioisotope atom per molecule of tracer. Other limitations not listed in Table 5 but stated by other investigators are the radiation hazards of the tracer used in the assay and the expense of sophisticated counting equipment. The first concern is minimal given the small amounts of radioisotopes routinely used in these assays, and the second concern is inappropriate because this instrumentation is available in most clinical laboratories performing routine assays. Moreover, the cost of this instrumentation has decreased with an increase in simplicity, efficiency (i.e., multiwell manual counters), and sophistication (data reduction equipment). Radioisotopes have not been used in homogeneous immunoassays because it is impossible to suppress radioisotope decay. Perhaps the most serious limitation to the use of radioisotopes is the concern regarding the disposal of the radioisotope. Decreasing hazardous landfill sites as well as increasing costs of disposal services have made the use of nonradioactive indicators more attractive. The major advantages that radioisotopes have over other indicators are the

Table 5. *The selection of an immunoassay indicator*

	Radioisotopes	Fluorophores	Enzymes
Advantages	Atomic size of indicator small Signal from tracer not affected by environment; no interference in reading signal Radioiodinate selective residues of protein No endogenous tracer in patient's serum	Atomic size of indicator small Long shelf life Preparation and purification of tracer simple Entire amount of indicator generates signal	Long shelf life Entire amount of indicator generates signal Signal occurs by amplification mechanism
Limitations	Limited shelf life Preparation and purification of tracer requires special facilities and experienced personnel Disposal of unincorporated radioisotope after preparation Only a fraction of indicator generates signal Decay catastrophe	Endogenous indicator in patient material Interference in reading signal of indicator from assay environment	May be endogenous indicator in patient material Interference in reading signal of indicator from assay environment Preparation and purification of tracer may be difficult Molecular size of indicator large

absence of interference in the production of a signal, the lack of endogenous indicator in the patient material, and the availability of a number of methods to radioiodinate proteins.

Fluorophores

The small atomic size, the long shelf-life, and the ease of measurement of fluorescent light make fluorophores desirable indicators for immunoassays. Most fluorophores can be covalently coupled to lysyl residues by reaction with the protein at alkaline pH. Purification of the tracer from uncoupled fluorophore is accomplished by dialysis or passage over a gel exclusion column. In addition, there is no concern about the cost and associated problems of radioactive waste disposal.

The major limitations of fluorophores as indicators are the presence of endogenous indicator in the patient material and interference in reading the signal of the indicator from the assay environment. For example, bilirubin and fluorescein isothiocyanate (FITC), the most widely used fluorophore in immunoassays, have similar spectral characteristics. Interfering substances in the assay may also absorb (i.e., quench) or scatter the fluorescent emission, which may compromise the accuracy of the assay. Lipid and other large molecules in the specimen will increase the scattering of fluorescent light, which in turn could decrease the detection of signal. One approach to minimizing the first and major limitation of fluorescent immunoassays is to read a "serum blank" for all specimens in the assay so that endogenous fluorescence in the specimen is subtracted from the measurement made in the assay. The other approach is to isolate the tracer from the endogenous fluorescence or interfering substances by making a high dilution of the specimen into the assay mixture or by performing immunometric (see below) or sandwich immunoassays where these substances can be removed by washing steps. However, in the latter immunoassays a careful choice of the solid phase support must be made so that similar problems are not acquired.

Enzymes

Enzymes potentially offer immunoassays the greatest degree of sensitivity because of the amplification that occurs when substrate is converted to product. The sensitivity can be increased substantially by measuring a fluorescent or radioactive product rather than a colorimetric product. However, a major problem encountered with this indicator and not with the others is the size of the enzyme molecule. Some of the coupling procedures used to link enzymes to either antigen or antibody may inactivate enzyme, antigen, or antibody. Moreover, some of the agents used in the conjugation procedure cross-link proteins nonspecifically so covalent linkage between like molecules often occurs. Thus, purification of the antibody-enzyme or antigen-enzyme tracer may be very difficult, and in some cases impossible. This problem is minimized by the use of two-step conjugation procedures. These procedures allow selective reaction with one reactant without cross-linking, followed by selective reaction with the other reactant, resulting in the production of an ideal tracer for enzyme immunoassay.

CHOICE OF IMMUNOASSAY METHOD

Assuming that one now has an appropriate antibody and suitable indicator, a decision must be made as to which type of immunoassay will provide the best assay system. Table 3 summarized the various types of assays that are routinely employed in clinical research. A detailed consideration of each will now be presented.

Competitive Saturation Immunoassays

The basic principle of the RIA initially described by Yalow and Berson was presented earlier. A diagrammatic representation of this assay is depicted in Fig. 1. Radioimmunoassays are classified as competitive saturation immunoassays because their basic feature is a competition in antigen excess between the unlabeled unknown or standard and a small amount of antigen indicator for binding to a limited number of antibody-combining sites. Fluorophores and enzymes have also been used as indicators in these assays. The major problems with using enzyme indicators are that the size of the molecule may alter or destroy crucial antigenic determinants that are recognized by high-affinity antibodies, the ideal enzyme-antigen conjugate cannot be prepared for every antigen because of the diversity in structure, and only a few bound and free separation procedures preserve enzymic activity.

The advantages and limitations of competitive saturation immunoassays are presented in Table 6. For two reasons these immunoassays are the most selective immunoassays that can be performed with polyclonal antisera. First, these assays use a restricted population of antibodies. The high dilution of antisera in the assay restricts reactivity of the antigen with high-affinity antibodies. This constraint sets a high threshold for generating a positive result and minimizes the possibility of cross-reactive or heteroclitic antibodies in low concentrations from binding antigen. Second, the specificity of the immune reaction is determined by the difference in affinity of the antibody for the homologous and heterologous determinant, since these reactions are run in extreme antigen excess. The sensitivity of these assays is limited by two major factors: (a) the affinity of the antibody as measured by an association constant and (b) the experimental error in the separation and measurement of the bound and free fractions. Further improvements in sensitivity can be achieved by increasing the affinity of the antibody, by minimizing the misclassification

TABLE 6. *Competitive saturation immunoassay*

Advantages	Limitations
1. Antibody population restricted	1. Antibody population restricted
2. Specificity proportional to difference in affinity	2. Sensitivity limited by association constant of antibody
3. Measure multivalent or univalent antigen	3. Sensitivity limited by separation of bound and free antigen
	4. Antigen-antibody reaction affected by environment
	5. Not easily adapted for enzyme immunoassay

error (i.e., correct reading of the indicator in the bound and free fractions), by delaying the addition of tracer to the assay, and by increasing the incubation time of the assay.

The use of a restricted population of antibodies may also be a limitation in two respects. First, high-affinity antibodies reacting against an inappropriate antigenic determinant may compromise the clinical utility of the assay because of unacceptable cross-reactivity. Adsorption of this antibody may result in antibody of lower affinity left in the antiserum, which in turn would decrease the sensitivity of the assay. Second, the reaction of high-affinity antibodies with antigen may be affected by substances in the patients' specimen or components in the assay mixture. The latter effect may be minimized by having the patient's specimen comprise 10% or less of the volume of the assay mixture.

Immunometric Immunoassays

The term *immunometric* was first used by Miles and Hale (6) to describe an immunoradiometric assay that used antibody indicator rather than antigen indicator as the tracer of the immune reaction. The antibody tracer is generally prepared by passage of the antiserum over an immunoadsorbent that contains the antigen. The antibody that binds to the adsorbent is radioiodinated and subsequently eluted of the absorbent. The assay is performed by incubating an excess amount of radiolabeled antibody with the standard or patients' specimen (Fig. 3A). Upon reaching equilibrium, solid phase particles containing the antigen are added to each tube and incubated for a short period. Quantitative determination of antigen is obtained by separating the soluble antigen-antibody

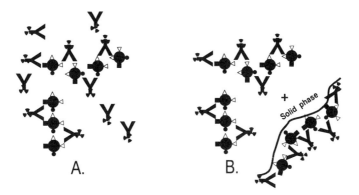

FIG. 3. Schematic of immunometric immunoassay demonstrating an excess of antibody-indicator binding antigen during initial incubation conditions (**A**) and the addition of solid phase carrying antigen to remove excess antibody indicator (**B**). In this assay, the supernatant solution is monitored for the indicator.

complexes from the insoluble antigen-antibody complex and counting the supernatant (Fig. 3B).

The advantages and limitations of immunometric immunoassay are presented in Table 7. The major advantage of these immunoassays is the assayability of antigens that are not easily labeled by an indicator molecule. Antibodies are very stable molecules with the same basic structure irrespective of specificity. A conjugation procedure developed for one antibody can be used for other antibodies from the same species or may only have to be modified slightly to be used for antibodies from other species. These assays can be easily adapted for the use of nonisotopic indicators. However, in these cases the antibody on the solid phase adsorbent is usually measured to minimize interference by endogenous tracer in the patient's specimen. Measurement of the solid phase particle also prolongs the lifetime of the tracer in immunoradiometric assays. Inactive antibody will not bind as antigen on the solid phase but will increase the background in the assay as originally described (6). Another modification that can be made in these assays is to use antiglobulin indicators to detect antibody bound to the solid phase.

The major limitation of these assays is the need for specifically purified antibody to prepare the tracer molecule. There are many problems associated with obtaining this type of reagent. First, the antibodies that are eluted off the immunoadsorbent column must be of the appropriate affinity. If the antibody indicator is of low affinity, it can dissociate from the soluble phase and attach to the solid phase antigen, compromising the sensitivity of the assay. The conditions used to elute the high-affinity antibodies off an immunoadsorbent can vary with antisera, requiring empiric determination of the appropriate

TABLE 7. *Immunometric immunoassay*

Advantages

- Allows performance of assays for antigens not easily labeled by indicator
- Uniform indicator coupling procedures can be developed
- Antibody indicator provides stable, long-lived tracer molecule
- Assay easily adapted for nonisotopic indicators
- Sensitivity not limited by association constant
- Assay of univalent or multivalent antigens

Limitations

- Specifically purified antibody often used as indicator
- Elution of purified antibody of appropriate affinity may be difficult
- Purified antigen needed for preparation of immunoadsorbents
- Wider diversity of antibody population
- Specificity determined by antibody avidity
- Antiglobulin antibody interferes with assay

---

elution conditions for each batch of antiserum. Second, the yield of antibody off the immunoadsorbent column is often suboptimal. Third, the harsh elution conditions that are used to elute high-affinity antibody often cause "stripping" of the antigen off the immunoadsorbent, which in turn contaminates the purified antibody preparation. Last, large amounts of purified antigen are needed for the immunoadsorbents that are used to prepare the specifically purified antibody and to separate the unreacted antibody in the assay.

The high concentrations of antibody used in these assays present other problems. First, antiglobulin antibodies in a patient's serum can act as a cross-linking agent to increase the amount of labeled antibody bound to the solid phase. Second, antibody excess assays are theoretically less specific than antigen excess assays because of the multivalent attachment of antibody to antigen and the increase in concentration of heteroclitic antibodies and of antibodies that cross-react with other antigens. Multivalent interaction can be eliminated by utilizing Fab fragments of the antibody in the assay.

Sandwich Immunoassay

The basic design of the sandwich immunoassay was outlined earlier and is depicted in Fig. 2. Three different variants in the design of this immunoassay can be performed. First, in the conventional sandwich immunoassay, antigen (i.e., patient's serum or standard) is initially incubated with the solid phase antibody, followed by a washing step, then incubation with antibody indicator, followed by an additional washing step with quantitative determination of the antibody indicator bound to the solid phase. Second, in the simultaneous sandwich immunoassay, all of the reagents are added at the initiation of the assay. Incubation is terminated by washing and counting the antibody indicator bound to the solid phase. In the third variant, the reverse sandwich immunoassay, antibody indicator is incubated initially with antigen followed by the addition of the solid phase antibody, which is used to separate antibody indicator-antigen complex from the free antibody indicator. Of these three, the 3-hour simultaneous sandwich assay is the least sensitive. The conventional sandwich assay increases the sensitivity of the assay approximately twofold but usually with an increase in the nonspecific binding in the assay. The reverse sandwich immunoassay is approximately three times more sensitive than the conventional assay with no further increase in nonspecific binding.

TABLE 8. *Sandwich immunoassay*
___

Advantages

- Allows performance of assays for antigens not easily labeled by indicator
- Uniform indicator coupling procedure can be developed
- Antibody indicator provides stable, long-lived tracer molecule
- Assay easily adapted for nonisotopic indicators
- Sensitivity not limited by association constant
- Antibody used to extract and to identify antigen-increase flexibility in assay and may increase resolution of antigen

Limitations

- Specifically purified antibody often used on solid phase as an indicator
- Elution of purified antibody of appropriate affinity may be difficult
- Purified antigen needed for preparation of immunoadsorbents
- Wider diversity of antibody population
- Specificity determined by antibody avidity
- Antiglobulin antibody interferes with assay
- Cannot measure univalent antigen
- High-dose hook effect
- Noncovalent attachment of antibody to solid phase may be unstable and/or irreproducible
___

TABLE 9. *Some important or interesting immunoassays arranged in groups*

Group[a]	Assay name	Acronym	Labels used[b]	Analytes[c]
1	Radio IA[d]	RIA	Radioisotopes	Unrestricted
	Chemilumino IA	CLIA	Chemiluminescent compounds	Unrestricted
	Enzymo IA	EIA	Enzymes	Unrestricted
	Fluoro IA	FIA	Fluorescent compounds	Unrestricted
2	Enzyme-linked immunosorbent assay	ELISA	Enzymes	Large antigens
	Immunochemilumino-metric assay compounds	ICLMA	Chemiluminescent	Large antigens
	Immunoradiometric assay	IRMA	^{125}I	Large antigens
3	Immunonephelometric assay		None	Large antigens
	Immunoturbidimetric assay		None	Large antigens
	Particle-enhanced turbidimetric inhibition IA	PETINIA	Latex particles	Large antigens
4	Enzyme-monitored IA technique	EMIT	GGPDH, MDH, lysozyme	Drugs and other haptens
	Fluorescence energy transfer IA	FETIA	2-Fluorescein derivatives	Immunoglobulin G
	Fluorescence polarization IA	PFIA	Fluorescein	Drugs and other haptens
	Substrate-labeled fluorescence IA	SLFIA	Umbelliferone	Theophylline

[a]See text for group criteria.
[b]General types of labeling substances cited for assay systems in widespread use.
[c]Individual analytes are cited if assay system not widely described in publications.
[d]IA = immunoassay

Sandwich immunoassays share many of the advantages and limitations of immunometric assays (Table 8) since both immunoassays are performed in antibody excess and often use specifically purified antibody for solid phase and antibody indicator reagents. The advantage these assays have over immunometric assays is that antibody rather than purified antigen is used on the solid phase. Antibodies are generally considered to be easier to purify and can be obtained in larger quantities than purified antigens. They also provide increased flexibility in the design of the immunoassay. Some limitations of sandwich immunoassays are that they cannot be used to measure covalent antigens and that high-dose hook effects in antibody indicator binding may be obtained with high concentrations of antigen in the patient's specimen. Another, more general, problem that can occur with any solid phase immunoassay is unstable or uneven coating of antigen or antibody to the solid phase. This problem is seen predominantly when antibody is used to passively coat plastic tubes or microtiter plates. The antibody binds noncovalently to the plastic by hydrophobic bonds which, during the course of an assay, can be destroyed, allowing antibody to come off the plastic. Likewise, other proteins in the assay system may bind to the plastic, leading to decreased sensitivity, increased background, and increased imprecision. To minimize these problems, plastic with the appropriate chemical composition must be used and the concentration of antibody used to coat the plate must be optimal to avoid layering of the protein on the plastic.

A summary of some important or interesting immunoassays is presented in Table 9. Included in this table are examples of competitive saturation immunoassays (Group 1), sandwich and immunometric immunoassays (Group 2),

TABLE 10. *Binding proteins used in immunoassays and related assays*

Binding protein		
Type or class	**Source**	**Analyte**
Binding proteins		
—Avidin	Chicken egg whites	Biotin
—B_{12} intrinsic factor	Porcine gastric mucosa	Vitamin B_{12}
—Lectin	Lotus$_{tetragonolobus}$	Haptoglobin
—Transcortin	Equine	Cortisol
Immunoglobulins		
—IgG polyclonal	Rabbit	Osteocalcin
	Chicken egg yolk	1,25-dihydroxyvitamin D
—IgG, F(ab')$_2$	Rabbit	hLH
—IgG, Fab'	Rabbit	Bovine LH
—IgG monoclonal	Mouse	HCG
	Rat	IgE antibody
—IgM monoclonal	Mouse	Tumor-associated antigen
Receptors	Synthetic	Teicoplanin
—Acyl-D-alanyl-D-alanine (binds vancomycin class antibiotics)		
—Receptor to γ-aminobutyric acid	Rat brain membrane	γ-aminobutyric acid
—Receptor to 1,25-dihydroxy-vitamin D	Calf thymus	1,25-dihydroxyvitamin D

precipitation or turbidimetric assays (Group 3), and other miscellaneous immunoassays, including those classified as homogeneous (Group 4). Although this listing is not inclusive, it does serve to highlight the utility and flexibility of these immunoassays.

Another assay system that can be used to quantitatively determine hormones is the radioreceptor assay. This assay is virtually identical to the competitive saturation immunoassay in that it is performed in antigen excess. However, no antibody is used. Rather, a preparation of the target cell hormone receptor protein is utilized as the binding protein. These assays can provide extremely high sensitivity, since many of the hormonal ligands are commercially available at very high specific activity. A major drawback to this assay is that the hormone usually must be isolated from the specimen and extensively purified before it can be quantitatively determined. In addition, many of the physiological receptors are quite labile, necessitating their preparation on a daily basis. A partial listing of binding proteins used in immunoassays and related assays can be found in Table 10.

HISTOLOGICAL TECHNIQUES

Many clinical research studies require laboratory techniques directed at assessing tissue histology. These methods are directed at quantitative determination of some physical change in the tissue or cellular properties and not necessarily at measuring the concentration of some analyte. Such techniques are very specialized and require the development of a dedicated histology laboratory. This task can be an expensive proposition when one considers the requirement for equipment such as microscopes and microtomes. In addition, the successful operation of such a facility will require experienced (a dying breed) or properly trained technicians proficient in the use and maintenance of such equipment. Again, the key to meaningful results with these histological methods is proper tissue handling and preparation.

Although the kinds of histological techniques available are as varied as the investigators who use them, most specimens must ultimately be examined by microscopy. The two general types of microscopy are (a) light microscopy and (b) electron microscopy. Each of these two categories is represented by specialized approaches, as summarized in Table 11.

Methods requiring light microscopy are pathological, morphometric, histochemical, immunohistological, and autoradiographic studies, to mention a few. Pathological studies generally examine tissue for evidence of abnormalities. Morphometric studies require measurements on the histological section of some abnormality such as cell number, scar area, or bone surface histology. Most of these measurements are performed with the assistance of appropriate electronic systems and software. Histochemical studies utilize some chemical property of the cells in that tissue and will stain selectively for those cells (property). On the other hand, immunohistochemical procedures require the use of an antigen-antibody reaction at the cell surface or at some cellular organelle. The antibody is usually tagged with a fluorescent dye so that cells manifesting antibody uptake can be readily seen under special light microscopic conditions. Finally, autoradiographic methods employ the use of a radioactive hormone, drug, or antibody, which is allowed to react with the tissue. Histological sections are prepared and placed next to photographic film. After weeks to months, the film is developed and the cellular location of the labeled material appears as discrete black dots.

Electron microscopy, on the other hand, can provide greater magnification and better resolution of the specimen under examination. However, because it employs a beam of electrons impinging on the specimen, special sample preparation techniques are required. Fixation in special solutions and carbon coating of the specimen surface to enhance resolution and to help conduct the build-up of electrical charge away from insulating and semi-insulating materials are required. Within the electron microscope family, there are two well-defined ranges of microscope, corresponding to transmission and reflection light microscopes, which examine directly the internal structure of translucent specimens and the outside features of bulk material, respectively.

The transmission electron microscope (TEM) is an obvious derivative of the compound light microscope, making use of the shorter wavelength electron illumination. In its simplest form it has exactly the same lens arrangement as its light counterpart. It has also been developed further to make fuller use of the

TABLE 11. *Partial list of histological techniques*

Light microscopy	Electron microscopy
Pathological	Pathological
Morphometric	Backscattered
Histochemical	Elemental analysis
Immunohistochemical	
Autoradiographic	

special properties of electron illumination—principally, the higher resolution, but also the ability to carry out various forms of elemental and crystallographic microanalysis. In its most powerful form it becomes the high-voltage electron microscope that uses electrons traveling at almost the speed of light to examine inside specimens that would be too thick for the normal TEM.

The electronic equivalent of the metallurgical or reflected light microscope, used to study the outside of materials rather than their internal arrangement, is the scanning electron microscope (SEM), whose ability to resolve fine detail lies intermediate between the light microscope and the high-resolution TEM. This instrument differs from all other microscopes using light or electrons in forming its image piecemeal and not all at one time. Its operation is dependent on a number of phenomena that occur at the sample surface under electron impact. Most important for scanning microscopy are the emission of secondary electrons with energies of a few tens of electron volts and re-emission or reflection of high-energy back-scattered electrons from the primary beam. The intensity of emission of both secondary and back-scattered electrons is very sensitive to the angle at which the electron beam strikes the surface (i.e., to topographical features on the specimen). The resolving power of SEM is on the order of 5 nm and can thus give a wealth of information about cellular histology. Recently, the back-scattered electron imaging technique has proven to be very useful in the assessment of new bone ingrowth on the surface of hydroxyapatite ceramic implants (3).

A close relative of the SEM is the scanning electron probe microanalyzer (EPMA). Instead of recording the scattered electrons, the microanalyzer records the emitted x-rays and sorts them according to wavelength by use of a special spectrophotometer. A quantitative analysis is made of a chemical element as the scanner picks up the distribution of the element. At the same time, an enlarged image may be displayed if the x-ray microspectrometer is part of a scanning electron microscopic system.

Increased use of the computer in conjunction with the EPMA has greatly improved the quality and quantity of the data obtained. Computers are now programmed to convert x-ray intensity ratios into chemical compositions and are now being used to automate repetitive EPMA analyses.

In addition to these techniques, additional methods such as field-emission microscopy and scanning acoustic microscopy have been reported (9,13). As previously mentioned, each of these specialized techniques will require its own particular sample requirements as well as sample preparatory methods. Success with these microscopic techniques can be facilitated by enlisting the help of experienced personnel. The high cost of the needed equipment for this type of clinical research generally restricts its location to pathology divisions where one can find experienced personnel to aid in the performance of these studies.

CELL CULTURE TECHNIQUES

The use of cell culture in clinical research has provided one of the most significant tools to understanding cellular physiology. Its applicability to clinical research, as well as its diversity, is exemplified by the types of studies that are possible with this technique. These studies include measurement of cellular proliferation and differentiation, hormone receptor characterization, and cellular actions of drugs, hormones, or growth factors. Moreover, cell culture can provide a source of DNA and RNA for molecular biological investigations.

The advantages and limitations of using cell culture in clinical research are summarized in Table 12. Examination of the cellular effects of various agents (e.g., drugs, growth factors) can be accomplished by direct addition of the agents *in vitro*. This is especially important in monitoring a biochemical event that could not be observed by *in vivo* or *in situ* techniques. Furthermore, because some control can be placed on cellular number and growth conditions, cell culture methods usually provide reproducible results within the same passage number. Although recombinant DNA techniques have proved to be of value in the provision of growth factors, hormones, and other biologically active substances, many of these agents are still purified from cells grown in culture and cell culture medium.

On the other hand, cell culture is expensive and time-consuming. Many of the culture medium additives, especially fetal calf serum, have become more limited in supply and thus more expensive to procure. Successful cell culture

TABLE 12. *Cell culture*

Advantages	Disadvantages
Permits study of cellular metabolism and response to external agents	Cells may not be passable
	Expensive and time-consuming
Provides concentrated source of material from which to isolate substances of interest (e.g., growth factors)	Cells may change phenotype during growth and passage
	Bacterial and/or fungal overgrowth
Usually provides reproducible results within same cell culture	Fibroblastic overgrowth
Cells can be used for histological studies	

techniques also require a technician who is well trained in the many facets of this method. Second, many of the cells used in culture may not be passable, necessitating experiments on a limited number of primary cells. Or worse, cells may undergo phenotypic changes in long-term culture requiring the establishment of a new primary cell line. This latter problem can be avoided by the use of transformed cell lines and by preparing frozen aliquots of the initial primary outgrowth of cells so that low-passage cultures can be restarted. Another disadvantage to cell culture is the potential for bacterial and/or fungal overgrowth in the culture medium, although this problem is usually nonexistent in a well-established and properly conducted cell culture facility.

The easiest way to establish a cell culture line is to try to obtain an established cell line from an outside source such as the American Type Culture Collection or from another investigator. Generally, these "starter" cultures will have been characterized with respect to their phenotype, thereby alleviating preliminary characterization experiments as well as establishing initial culture conditions. If such a cell type is not available as a nontransformed cell line, one should consider the use of a transformed cell line. Transformed cell lines generally grow rapidly in culture and can provide a large number of cells for the intended studies. The phenotype of transformed cells should be identical to that of the nontransformed cell type being used. However, many of the responses of transformed cells may be greatly augmented or suppressed as compared to the normal cell, suggesting to some investigators that results from *in vitro* studies in transformed cells should be cautiously extended to the situation found in normal cells.

If a previously established cell line (normal or transformed) is not available, one must consider preparation of the cells from tissue. For blood cells, this task is relatively simple, involving centrifugation through special gradients such as Ficoll-Hypaque. This procedure will yield an enriched population of cells (e.g., lymphocytes) with little contamination from other cell types. This enriched cell population can then be transferred to culture or immortalized by viral infection to yield a population of cells that can be used repeatedly in molecular biology studies. If the starting tissue is soft or hard, a different approach must be used. The simplest approach is to chop the tissue into small fragments and to culture the tissue pieces in the appropriate medium. The goal of this technique is to procure the appropriate cell type as a primary outgrowth from the tissue explants. This approach has been successfully used for bone tissue to obtain an enriched population of osteoblasts. This procedure is time-consuming, requiring 3 to 4 weeks to obtain a confluent primary outgrowth. It is also limited by the potential of growing a mixed cell population. For example, the primary outgrowth of osteoblasts from bone chips may also contain fibroblastic cells. This secondary cell growth can be minimized in part by performing an initial

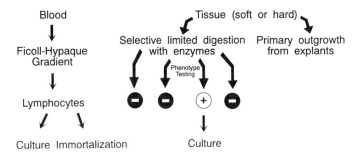

FIG. 4. Flow chart for the preparation of cells for culture from various tissue types.

selective limited digestion of the tissue with enzymes to remove the contaminating cell population. This task is usually accomplished by collecting the various populations of cells released at each digestion step, plating the cells, and testing for the appropriate phenotype to ascertain which population of released cells comprises the desired cell type. Another option is to vary the culture conditions by substituting culture media that will promote the growth of only the cell type in question. A summary of these considerations is presented in Fig. 4. A more detailed approach to basic cell culture can be found in various instructional manuals (1,7).

REFERENCES

1. Freshney, R.I., editor (1987): *Culture of Animal Cells: A Manual of Basic Techniques.* Alan R. Liss, New York.
2. Gosling, J.P. (1990): A decade of development in immunoassay methodology. *Clin. Chem.* 36:1408–1427.
3. Holmes, R.E., Hagler, H.K., and Coletta, C.A. (1987): Thick-section histometry of porous hydroxyapatite implants using backscattered electron imaging. *J. Biomed. Mater. Res.* 21:731–739.
4. Kohler, G. and Milstein, C. (1975): Continuous cultures of fused cells secreting antibody of predefined specificity. *Nature* 256:495–497.
5. McCarthy, R.C. (1985): Basic concepts in antibody recognition: implications for immunoassay of multivalent antigens. In:*Clinical Laboratory Annual,* edited by H.A. Homburger and J.G. Batsakis, pp. 65–104. Appleton-Century-Crofts, Norwalk, CT.
6. Miles, L.E.M. and Hale C.N. (1968): Labelled antibodies and immunological assay systems. *Nature* 219:186–189.
7. Pollard, J.W. and Walker, J.M., editors (1990): *Methods in Molecular Biology. 5: Animal Cell Culture.* Humana Press, Clifton, NJ.

8. Reckhel, R. (1989): Monoclonal antibodies: clinical applications. In: *Advances in Clinical Chemistry*, edited by H.E. Spiegel, pp. 355–415. Academic Press, San Diego.
9. Rochow, T.G. and Rochow, E.G., editors. (1978): *An Introduction to Microscopy by Means of Light, Electrons, X-rays, or Ultrasound*. Plenum Press, New York.
10. Siest, G., Henny, J., Schiele, F., and Young, D.S., editors. (1985): *Interpretation of Clinical Laboratory Tests: Reference Values and Their Biological Variation*. Biomedical Publications, Foster City, CA.
11. Solberg, H.E. and Grasbeck, R. (1989): Reference values. In: *Advances in Clinical Chemistry*, edited by H.E. Spiegel, pp. 1–79. Academic Press, San Diego.
12. Vetterlein, D. (1989): Monoclonal antibodies: production, purification, and technology. In: *Advances in Clinical Chemistry*, edited by H.E. Spiegel, pp. 303–354. Academic Press, San Diego.
13. Watt, I.M., editor (1985): *The Principles and Practice of Electron Microscopy*. Cambridge University Press, Cambridge.
14. Yalow, R.S. and Berson, S.A. (1959): Assay of plasma insulin in human subjects by immunological methods. *Nature* 184:1648–1649.

8

The Metabolic Balance Regimen and the Nutritional Aspects of Clinical Research

Linda Brinkley and Charles Y. C. Pak

Center for Mineral Metabolism and Clinical Research, University of Texas Southwestern Medical Center at Dallas, Dallas, Texas 75235-8885

Nutrition could play a critical role in clinical research in two ways. First, a nutritional problem may be the primary focus of clinical research. Such a primary nutritional research might be exemplified by the examination of a high monounsaturated diet on cholesterol control (8) or the effect of animal protein diet on the propensity for kidney stone formation (4).

More commonly, nutrition plays an ancillary role in clinical research. Dietary aberrations could alter serum and urinary biochemistry and modify physiological presentation. By imposing a constant dietary regimen, the "true" metabolic status may be discerned without interference by dietary influences. For example, a controlled sodium intake is critical in examining the renin-angiotensin system and aldosterone secretion (9). A constant diet with fixed intakes of calcium, phosphorus, and sodium is required in differentiating various forms of hypercalciuria (19).

The degree of dietary control is dependent on specific requirements of the study. The classic full metabolic balance represents the most rigid form of dietary control. Because of its complexity and great demand on commitment and time, it is being replaced by less rigorous dietary measures of shorter duration. For example, dietary control may be accomplished by use of constant frozen diets in an outpatient setting, and information previously derived from the state of balance of a particular nutrient may be sought by other, simpler means.

It is our objective in this chapter to review the principles, applications, and conduct of metabolic balance studies. Simpler forms of dietary control will then be described. The chapter concludes with a discussion of often ignored but important principles of nutritional aspects of clinical research—bioavailability and drug-nutrient and nutrient-nutrient interactions.

THE CLASSIC METABOLIC BALANCE TECHNIQUE

Definition

Metabolic balance defines the net gain or deficit of a particular nutrient or nutrients. It is determined by analysis of the nutrient in question in the diet, urine, and feces. The balance is said to be positive when the dietary content of the nutrient exceeds the loss in urine and feces. Conversely, the balance is negative if losses in urine and feces exceed the dietary intake. The balance is zero when the losses equal the intake.

The Essential Elements of Metabolic Balance

The objective of the metabolic balance approach is to control the environment as much as possible so that findings observed can be attributed to the underlying disease process or to a particular procedure or medication under study. The technique's reliability depends on the provision of an isocaloric constant diet with desired composition and fixed fluid intake, stabilization on the diet, accurate urine and fecal collection, and control of physical activity and stresses. Because of its rigorous demands, metabolic balance study can best be done in the setting of the general clinical research center equipped with a metabolic kitchen and a routine core laboratory.

The Provision of an Isocaloric Constant Diet

It is the basic function of the research center kitchen staff to control the intake of food and fluids of study subjects (28). Teamwork and accuracy are absolute requirements. Specific and detailed procedures for measuring, preparing, and serving daily food and fluids must be defined and followed. Exact procedures are established to eliminate the loss of food or fluid until it is consumed by subjects. A cooperative attitude on the part of the members of the research team and the commitment of each in carrying out the many details of the prescribed procedure are essential to success (25).

The Types of Constant Diets

A *liquid formula diet* offers the most rigid control and can be chemically designed to accommodate many different types of nutritional studies (2). Because of the ease of preparation, ingredient costs may be less and fewer staff are needed (13). Other advantages are constancy of composition and the need for minimal storage space. However, the liquid formula diet may be acceptable to patients for only short periods; usual complaints are monotony and having nothing to chew. In addition, the low residue content may reduce stool volume or result in constipation. Conversely, the nutrient density of the liquid diet may cause diarrhea and/or nausea.

The *24-hour menu* is a three- to six-meal plan of solid food that is repeated daily without variation for the duration of the study (28). This plan is advantageous because preparing and serving the same diet day after day minimizes the chance of error and requires less work on the part of laboratory and kitchen staff. It permits a normal fashion of eating solid foods, as opposed to drinking fluids with the liquid formula, and is, therefore, more readily accepted. Metabolic balance studies of short-to-moderate duration often utilize this type of diet plan because of the accuracy provided by the unchanging nature of the daily diet. However, this plan may not be suitable for long-term studies due to its repetitive nature.

The *rotation diet plan* comprises a series of two to five daily menus that are of similar nutrient composition but offer diverse foods. Once the menus are calculated and agreed to by the patient, the composition and the rotation of different daily menus remain the same throughout the study. This plan offers the subject greater variety and is, therefore, often used in studies of long duration.

However, the rotation diet plan has disadvantages of greater chance for error and more workload for the nutrition and laboratory staff.

Diet selection depends on the needs of the study and its length, the emotional and physiological tolerance of the patient, the facilities of the laboratory and kitchen, and the philosophy of the investigator. The investigator and the dietitian should be in agreement about the most efficient and successful way to achieve desired study results (7).

All food is weighed by electronic scale or measured by graduated cylinder and cooked for each patient individually. Food is purchased in processing batch lots, weighed raw, and then cooked without losing anything during the cooking process (28).

The Interview with a Dietitian

Once a person has been selected to undergo a study, it is vital that the dietitian, as well as other members of the research team, orient the patient to the techniques and procedures that will be required. The importance of the nutrition interview cannot be overemphasized. Dietary problems are less likely to occur when adequate planning, time, and attention are devoted to this interview. In addition to the patient's food preferences, other dietary factors may need to be considered. For example, a patient undergoing a study of calcium metabolism may also have diabetes, be a vegetarian, have lactose intolerance, or require a low-fat low-cholesterol modification. The nutrition interview can ascertain these needs and, with that information, the dietitian can accommodate these special needs during diet calculation.

Although diets should be developed around the patient's personal eating pattern, experience indicates that bland foods are best tolerated when the same diet is repeated day after day. Generally, beef and/or chicken breast are better accepted than other meats. However, ground lamb, ground veal, and ground pork are also satisfactory if lean and thoroughly mixed. The cellulose husk of corn kernels may act as a barrier to digestion; therefore, if corn is used, it must be blended. Foods that may confuse or complicate dietary calculation or study interpretation might be omitted. In the study of calcium absorption, the use of spinach, rhubarb, chocolate, or oatmeal might be limited because their content of oxalate or phytate may bind calcium. The red color of beets may interfere with certain laboratory analyses (creatinine) or fecal marker recognition (28).

The Problem of Incomplete Food Consumption

Since it is essential to the success of the study, every effort must be made to assure that the patients consume all of their food. However, rejection of food due to illness or spillage can occur. The procedure for handling this problem should be established in advance. Thus, the nutrient content of refused food can be calculated and replaced if possible, refused food can be saved and presented to the patient later in the 24-hour period, or rejected food can be analyzed and the composition noted in the chart to explain any variation in results on that particular day.

Spilled food that affects the accuracy of the patient's intake must be reported as an error. If possible, spilled food should be recovered, weighed, and sent to the laboratory for analysis (28).

Stabilization on the Diet

Before a formal metabolic balance begins, patients must be stabilized on the specified metabolic diet. In general, it requires about 4 days for a steady-state status to be reached for calcium balance, 4 to 6 days for sodium balance, and about 2 weeks for lipid balance (Fig. 1). Large errors could result if the metabolic balance study is begun prematurely, as it would include erroneous data.

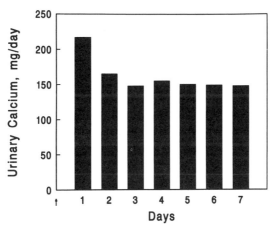

FIG. 1. Stabilization on a metabolic diet, begun on Day 0, as indicated by the *arrow*.

Accurate Urine and Fecal Collection

The reliability of metabolic balance depends on accurate urine and fecal collection, as well as precise measurement of desired constituents in urine, feces, and diet.

Urine Collection

All urine samples must be collected in 24-hour pools throughout the study period. Patients should be instructed to begin collection at a precise time (e.g., at 8 a.m. to coincide with breakfast) and to close exactly 24-h later each day. The first void at the beginning of collection on Day 1 is to be discarded. In each day, all subsequent voids are to be saved, with care given to empty the bladder completely exactly 24 hours later.

The accuracy of urine collection may be estimated from urinary creatinine. In normal men, urine creatinine averages 21 mg/kg, whereas the mean value in normal women is 17 mg/kg.

Fecal Collection

Because of the delay in intestinal transit, stool specimens collected on a given day do not generally correspond to urine specimens obtained or meals ingested on that same day, but lag behind by one to several days. Thus, fecal "marking" is necessary. In one approach (20), a "period marker" such as carmine or charcoal is given at bedtime of the evening before the beginning of the study period and repeated every 4 days, marking the end of each 4-day period. Moreover, a continuous marker such as polyethylene glycol is given daily during stabilization, study periods, and the poststudy period until the appearance of the last period marker.

All fecal specimens are collected separately at each void, with the exact time and date marked on the containers. Specimens showing visible period marker would be identified (carmine red or charcoal black). Specimens between two markers would be pooled, such that collections between the first and the second markers would correspond to Period 1, collections between the second and the third markers would represent Period 2, and so on.

Each fecal pool corresponding to each 4-day study period would be homogenized and analyzed for polyethylene glycol. From the recovery of this nonabsorbable marker in feces, a correction can be made for the accuracy of fecal collection.

Diet Analysis

If a 24-hour menu is utilized, a duplicate of the patient's food and fluid intake for one whole day is homogenized and analyzed for desired nutrient content. When the rotation diet plan is used, all daily menus must be analyzed.

The Control of Physical Activity and Stresses

The objective of the metabolic regimen is to stabilize patients in an environment free of external stresses so as to expose the underlying metabolic state. Thus, strenuous physical activity, extremes of ambient temperature, and emotionally stressful confrontation should be avoided. Nonstudy medications that are not critical to maintenance of health should be withdrawn if possible.

It is advisable to restrict passes to outside the hospital during metabolic dietary regimen. In a common case, urinary chemistry, obtained from a patient given a pass, disclosed lower urinary sodium, pH, and volume on the day of the pass. The patient admitted to running outside despite caution to remain indoors in air-conditioned areas.

An Illustration of a Metabolic Balance Study

The classic calcium balance technique was used to elucidate the mechanism of action of sodium cellulose phosphate in nephrolithiasis due to absorptive hypercalciuria (18) (Fig. 2). Before treatment, urinary calcium was high and fecal calcium low, suggesting that hypercalciuria originated from an intestinal hyperabsorption of calcium. After therapy with sodium cellulose phosphate, urinary calcium decreased by one-half as fecal calcium doubled. The results indicated that this drug reduced intestinal calcium absorption by binding calcium, thereby restoring normal urinary calcium.

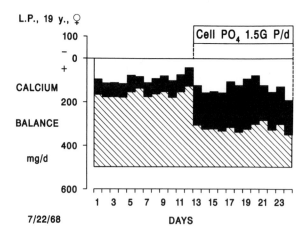

FIG. 2. Effect of sodium cellulose phosphate on calcium balance. The calcium balance was plotted as follows. The intake line was plotted downward from the zero line. Urinary calcium is shown above the intake line as the *hatched areas,* and fecal calcium by *shaded areas.* The *clear area* below the zero line represents the extent of positive calcium balance. During cellulose phosphate therapy, urinary calcium decreased by approximately 50% and fecal calcium increased approximately twofold.

During both control and treatment periods, the sum of urinary and fecal calcium was less than the dietary calcium intake. Thus, the patient was in positive calcium balance treatment and remained so despite inhibition of calcium absorption by sodium cellulose phosphate treatment.

THE MODIFIED METABOLIC DIETARY REGIMEN

Classic metabolic balance studies are infrequently utilized now. They have been replaced by a short-term constant dietary regimen without fecal collection, where the patient's metabolic status is assessed by simpler measures, such as the concentration in blood and urinary excretion of implicated hormones or metabolites. A constant diet is then used to help control the environment, so that the underlying physiological-metabolic status or disturbances can be identified. Overall requirements are, therefore, not as rigid as in the classic metabolic balance study. Some of the allowable modifications are described below.

Food Composition Tables

When facilities for food analysis are limited or nonexistent, metabolic diets may be calculated using data from food composition tables or nutrient database software programs. However, there are drawbacks. The major problem with available tables and databases is missing data. Nutrients such as oxalate, sulfur, or purine are often omitted (22). Whole sections of analyses, such as those for fatty acids or amino acids, may be missing. Another problem is the differences in reported food composition among various sources. This problem may be due to inconsistencies in analytical methods. There may also be variations in composition due to the type of feed and fertilizer, climate, soil composition, and processing techniques. The best and most complete food composition information is available from the U.S. Department of Agriculture (27).

The diversity of food components is vast. Of the naturally occurring components, energy-providing nutrients, essential nutrients, and dietary fiber can usually be found in nutrient databases. However, food composition of natural toxins such as the goitrogens found in some edible roots and leaves, antinutrient substances such as the biotin antagonist avidin, and other naturally occurring compounds such as DNA, RNA, enzymes, sterols, and caffeine may be more difficult to find. Amounts of intentional food additives such as salt and seasonings may be found, but information on agricultural additives such as pesticides may not be available. Analyses of microbial and fungal toxins and parasites, inadvertent additives such as leached metals and iodide, and compounds formed in food processing, storage, and preparation may not be available. Complete analytical information on new engineered and designer foods such as foods using fat substitutes or sugar substitutes may not be available (15).

Many journals are now recommending that data generated from a nutrient database be cited, giving the name of the database, the software developer and trade name, the copyright year and the year of most recent update, the version number (if available), and a description of modifications or additions to the database.

Frozen Metabolic Diets

Frozen metabolic diets are made up of metabolic meals, quickly frozen immediately after preparation, which are designed for use in an outpatient setting. Standard frozen metabolic diets of fixed caloric contents (1,500, 2,000, or 2,500 calories/day), offered to patients without prior choice or selection, are particularly useful for short-term studies. For longer use, frozen diets may be designed for each patient after a personal nutrition interview.

Frozen metabolic diets may reduce the need for inpatient hospitalization, since they may be used for stabilization in an outpatient setting and as an entire study may be carried out using them in an ambulatory setting. However, careful instruction and monitoring of patients and selection of reliable patients are critical.

OTHER NUTRITIONAL CONSIDERATIONS

Bioavailability

Bioavailability is the amount of nutrient that is actually available for absorption and utilization from food. It is a factor that is often ignored in nutrition. In nutritional tables, for example, the total amount of a nutrient is typically given among various food items. There is an implicit assumption that the specified nutrient is equally bioavailable from all food sources. Unfortunately, such is not the case for many nutrients.

Magnesium and zinc absorption may be decreased in the presence of phytate and fiber in the diet. The best sources of biotin are liver, egg yolk, soy flour, cereals, and yeast, but the bioavailability varies considerably depending upon whether it is present in an unbound form (as it is in most foods) or in a bound form (as in wheat). In general, free fluoride as it exists in water is more available for absorption than is the protein-bound fluorine in foods. Different forms of folate vary in stability under various conditions but, in general, heat, oxidation, and ultraviolet light may cleave the folate molecule, rendering it inactive. As much as 50% of food folate may be destroyed during household preparation, food processing, and storage. With few exceptions, nutrients in a readily bioavailable form are present in human milk in proportions appropriate for adequate nutrition for the first 3 to 6 months of life. However, infants absorb 65% to 70% of the phosphorus in cow's milk and 85% to 90% of that in human milk. Niacin, which is found in high concentrations in meats, is stable in foods and can withstand reasonable periods of heating, cooking, and storage with little loss. However, in some foods, such as cereal grains, as much as 70% of the niacin may be biologically unavailable because of the structure of the compounds in which it is bound (5).

In cereal-based foods, niacin bioavailability is poor unless treated with lime. The bioavailability of zinc in foods varies widely. Meat, liver, eggs, and seafood (especially oysters) are good sources of available zinc, whereas whole grain products contain the element in a less available form (17).

The disparity between calcium content and absorbed calcium is shown in Table 1. Spinach is a rich source of calcium, but the high oxalate content of the spinach binds the calcium, making it largely unavailable for absorption. Thus, despite a high calcium content of 380 mg/200-g serving, only 8.4 mg is absorbed from the gastrointestinal tract. However, the calcium bioavailability from milk chocolate is much higher. While 90 g of milk chocolate contains a modest amount of calcium (216 mg), the amount of absorbed calcium is much higher than that from spinach (21.8 mg) (5).

Food-Drug Interactions

Drug therapy can affect nutritional status by altering food intake or absorption, metabolism, and the excretion of nutrients (3). On the other hand, food intake can alter the absorption, metabolism, and excretion of certain drugs.

TABLE 1. *Calcium-content and bioavailability*

Food item	Calcium content (mg)	Bioavailability	Absorbed calcium (mg)
Spinach (200 g)	380	2.2%	8.4
Turnip greens (200 g)	360	5.1%	18.4
Tea, brewed (10 g tea in 250 ml dist. water plus 250 ml milk)	310	5.3%	16.4
Okra (200 g)	280	2.3%	6.4
Milk chocolate (90 g)	216	10.1%	21.8
Almonds (100 g)	190	2.8%	5.3
Peanuts (100 g)	116	13.7%	15.9
V-8 juice (500 ml)	75	10.1%	7.6
Orange juice (500 ml)	65	10.5%	6.8
Pecans (60 g)	42	32.6%	13.7
Cranberry juice (500 ml)	30	31.3%	9.4
Tea, instant (10 g)	10	100.0%	10.0
Tea, brewed (10 g in 500 ml dist. water)	10	50.1%	5.0

Awareness of these potential interactions can help prevent nutrient deficiencies and impairment or exaggeration of the drug action (10). These considerations emphasize the need to withhold nonessential drugs during metabolic studies.

The following tables describe various forms of food-drug interactions. Certain drugs may depress or enhance appetite (Table 2) (14). Others may alter food intake by affecting taste sensitivity (Table 3) (6,24). Some foods can affect the action of certain drugs by impairing or enhancing their gastrointestinal absorption, providing factors that alter drug action, or creating an environment that influences drug activity (Table 4) (10). Some drugs may affect nutrient availability (Table 5) (3).

Nutrient-Nutrient Interactions

Certain nutrients can affect the availability or absorption of others. However, these interactions may have opposing effects on different organ systems. A high-fiber diet has been suggested to be useful in cholesterol control (29) and in the prevention of colon cancer (16). However, it may impair the absorption of calcium due to its high content of phytate, which is capable of binding calcium (12). Citrus fruit juices may improve the absorbability of calcium from sparingly soluble calcium salts such as calcium carbonate by forming a more

TABLE 2. *Drugs that affect appetite*

Appetite depressants	Appetite stimulants
Amphetamines and related compounds	Antidepressants
—Benzphetamine (Didrex)	Amitriptyline (Elavil)
—Fenfluramine (Pondimin)	Cyproheptadine (Periactin)
—Phenmetrazine (Preludin)	Lithium carbonate (Lithane)
—Phenylpropanolamine	Minor tranquilizers
(Dexatrim, Dimetapp, Triaminic)	—Benzodiazepines (Clonopin,
Antibiotics	Valium)
—Amphotericin B (Fungizone)	—Phenothiazines (Phenergan)
—Gentamicin (Garamycin)	Major tranquilizers
Carbonic anhydrase inhibitors	—Chlorpromazine (Thorazine)
—Acetazolamide (Diamox)	Steroids
—Dichlorphenamide (Daranide)	—Anabolic steroids (Anavar)
Digitalis preparations	—Glucocorticoids (Decadron,
Methylphenidate (Ritalin)	Medrol)
	—Tetrahydrocannabinol (marijuana)

TABLE 3. *Drugs that affect taste sensitivity*

Amphetamines (↓ sweet, ↑ bitter)	Lincomycin
Ampicillin	Lithium carbonate (strange
Amphotericin B	unpleasant taste)
Aspirin	Meprobamate
Captopril	Metronidazole
Chlorpheniramine maleate	Methicillin (aftertaste)
Clindamycin (bitter aftertaste)	Oxyfedrine
Clofibrate (↓ sensitivity, aftertaste)	Penicillamine
Diazoxide	Phenindione
Dinitrophenol	Phenytoin
Ethancrynic acid	Propantheline
Griseofulvin	Sodium lauryl sulfate
Insulin	Streptomycin
	Tetracyclines

Sensitivity is decreased except for increased bitterness with amphetamine

TABLE 4. *Foods and nutrients that could alter drug action*

Food	Effect	Drug	Mechanism
Alkalinizing foods	↓	Methenamine	Urinary alkalinization
	↑	Quinidine	Enhanced absorption
	↑	Quinine	Enhanced absorption
Caffeine	↑	Theophylline	Drug potentiation
Fatty foods	↑	Griseofulvin	Enhanced absorption
High fiber foods	↓	Digoxin	Impaired absorption
Licorice	↓	Antihypertensive agents	Provision of salt-retaining sterol
	↓	Digitalis	Provision of salt-retaining sterol
Milk and dairy products	↓	Tetracycline	Impaired absorption
Low-salt diet	↑	Lithium	Enhanced absorption
High-salt diet	↓	Lithium	Impaired absorption
Tyramine-containing foods	↑	MA01 antidepressants	Drug potentiation
Vitamin K-rich foods	↓	Anticoagulants	Antagonism
Foods rich in Fe, Ca, or Zn	↓	Tetracycline	Impaired absorption

TABLE 5. *Drugs that can affect nutrient availability*

Drug	Effect	Nutrient
Antacids	↓	Vit A & B, Fe
Barbiturates	↓	Iron
Ca phosphate	↓	Iron
Cholestyramine	↓	Vit A & D
Mineral oil	↓	Vit A, D, E, & K
Penicillamine	↓	Cu, Zn, Fe
Primidone	↓	Folic acid
Sulfasalazine	↓	Folic acid

soluble calcium citrate (23). However, they may cause aluminum retention when given to patients with end-stage renal disease with aluminum-containing antacids by stimulating the formation of absorbable aluminum-citrate complex (26). Ascorbic acid has been touted for various health claims, including the prevention of colds (21). However, it may produce hyperoxaluria (11), increasing the risk for kidney stone formation. These opposing interactions should be carefully considered before recommending any dietary program.

The Effect of Biotechnology on Nutrition

Biotechnology could have an influence on future food composition and nutrient intake (1). Techniques of genetic engineering have been applied to plants, animals, and microorganisms to enhance the nutritional quality of food and to improve food safety. This approach will undoubtedly open new areas of research regarding nutrient composition, digestion, and absorption. Table 6 lists various uses of genetic engineering in plants and animals. At present, the Food and Drug Administration does not have guidelines regarding the use or approval of genetically engineered foods.

SUMMARY

Clinical research often requires dietary control in the study of the underlying physiological or metabolic status of patients. Under such a controlled setting, the effect of an intervention (drug) or the pathophysiology of the disease

TABLE 6. *Uses of genetic engineering in nutrition*

 1. Attainment of desired ratio of amino acids in grain products
 2. Enhancement of soluble fiber content
 3. Alteration of fatty acid composition of oils
 4. Reduction in fat and cholesterol content
 5. Reduction in calorie content
 6. Enrichment with antioxidants
 7. Enhancement with vitamins and minerals
 8. Enhancement of nutrient density
 9. Development of resistance to spoilage or insect damage
10. Inhibition of caffeine production in coffee plants

process can be better elucidated. The classic metabolic balance technique is infrequently used today, with the introduction of more sophisticated techniques of assessing metabolic or hormonal status. However, a controlled metabolic dietary regimen, albeit without a full balance, is still critical in many clinical research studies.

Factors such as food composition, nutrient bioavailability, and food-drug interactions may influence the outcome of some clinical studies and therefore must be taken into consideration. Nutrition is often important in the design and implementation of well-controlled studies that address questions relevant to human health.

REFERENCES

1. Adler, J. and Denworth, L. (1992): Splashing in the gene pool. *Newsweek,* March 9:71.
2. Ahrens, E.H. (1970): The use of liquid formula diets in metabolic studies: 15 years experience. *Adv. Metab. Disorders* 4:297–332.
3. American Medical Association (1980): *AMA Drug Evaluations. 4th ed.* AMA Department of Drugs, Chicago.
4. Breslau, N.A., Brinkley, L., Hill, K.D., and Pak, C.Y.C. (1988): Relationship of animal protein-rich diet to kidney stone formation and calcium metabolism. *J. Clin. Endocrinol. Metab.* 66:140–146.
5. Brinkley, L.J., McGuire, J., Gregory, J., and Pak, C.Y.C. (1981): Bioavailability of oxalate in foods. *Urology* 17:534–538.
6. Carson, J.A.S. and Gormican, A. (1976): Disease-medication relationships in altered taste sensitivity. *J. Am. Diet. Assoc.* 68:550.
7. De St. Jeor, S.T. and Bryan, G.T. (1973): Clinical research diets: definition of terms. *J. Am. Diet. Assoc.* 62:47–50.
8. Garg, A., Bonanome, A., Grundy, S.M., Zhang, Z.J., and Unger, R.H. (1988): Comparison of a high-carbohydrate diet with high-monounsaturated-fat diet in patients with non-insulin-dependent diabetes mellitus. *N. Engl. J. Med.* 319:829–834.

9. Gomez-Sanchez, C.E. and Holland, O.B. (1981): Urinary tetrahydroaldosterone and aldosterone-18-glucuronide excretion in white and black normal subjects and hypertensive patients. *J. Clin. Endocrinol. Metab.* 52:214–219.

10. Harkness, R. (1984): *Drug Interactions Handbook.* Prentice-Hall, Englewood Cliffs, NJ.

11. Hellman, L. and Burns, J.J. (1958): Metabolism of L-ascorbic acid 1-C^{14} in man. *J. Biol. Chem.* 230:923–930.

12. Kelsay, J.L. (1982): Effects of fiber on mineral and vitamin bioavailability. In: *Dietary Fiber in Health & Disease,* edited by G.V. Vahouny and D. Kritchevsky. Plenum Press, New York.

13. King, J.C. and Calloway, D.H. (1969): The cost of research diets. *J. Am. Diet. Assoc.* 55:361–365.

14. Levitsky, D.A. (1984): Drugs, appetite and body weight. In: *Drugs and Nutrients: The Interactive Effects,* edited by D.A. Roe and T.C. Campbell. Marcel Dekker, New York.

15. Monsen, E.R. (1991): Nutrient database for the 90's: excellence in diversity. Presented at the 16th National Nutrient Databank Conference, San Francisco, June 17–19, 1991.[1]

16. National Research Council (1989a): Diet and health: implications for reducing chronic disease risk. In: *Report of the Committee on Diet & Health, Food and Nutrition Board.* National Academy Press, Washington, DC.

17. National Research Council (1989b): *Recommended Dietary Allowances.* 10th ed. National Academy Press, Washington, DC.

18. Pak, C.Y.C. (1973): Sodium cellulose phosphate: mechanism of action and effect on mineral metabolism. *J. Clin. Pharmacol.* 13:15–27.

19. Pak, C.Y.C., Ohata, M., Lawrence, E.C., and Snyder, W. (1974): The hypercalciurias: causes, parathyroid functions and diagnostic criteria. *J. Clin. Invest.* 54:387–400.

20. Pak, C.Y.C., Stewart, A., Raskin, P., and Galosy, R.A. (1980): A simple and reliable method for calcium balance using combined period and continuous fecal markers. *Metabolism* 29:793–798.

21. Pauling, L. (1971): The significance of the evidence about ascorbic acid and the common cold. *Proc. Natl. Acad. Sci. USA* 68:2678–2681.

22. Pennington, J.A.T. (1989): *Food Values of Portions Commonly Used.* 15th ed. Harper & Row, Publishers, New York.

23. Recker, R.R. (1985): Calcium absorption and achlorhydria. *N. Engl. J. Med.* 313:70–73.

24. Roe, D.A. (1979): Interactions between drugs and nutrients. *Med. Clin. North Am.* 63:985.

25. Sampson, A.G., Sprague, A.G., and Wollaeger, E.E. (1952): Dietary techniques for metabolic balance studies. *J. Am. Diet. Assoc.* 28:912–915.

26. Slanina, P., Frech, W., Skostrom, L., Loof, L., Slorach, S., and Cedergren, A. (1986): Dietary citric acid enhances absorption of aluminum in antacids. *Clin. Chem.* 32:539–541.

27. U.S. Department of Agriculture (1976): *Composition of Foods.* Agriculture Handbook No.8. Agricultural Research Service, Washington, DC.

28. U.S. Department of Health, Education and Welfare, National Institutes of Health (1969): *A Dietetic Manual for Metabolic Kitchen Units.* Nutrition Department, Clinical Center, Bethesda, MD.

29. Vahouny, G.V. (1982): Dietary fiber, lipid metabolism and atherosclerosis. *Fed. Proc.* 41:2801–2806.

9

The Role of the General Clinical Research Center in Clinical Research

Neil A. Breslau, M.D.

*Department of Medicine, University of Texas Southwestern Medical Center
at Dallas, Dallas, Texas 75235*

As an endocrinology fellow at Upstate Medical Center in Syracuse, I frequently passed a building upon which the following quotation was inscribed: "Dedicated to those of scientific mind and investigative spirit who purpose to serve humanity." These words succinctly describe the role of the General Clinical Research Center Program. The GCRCs offer a research infrastructure, often otherwise unavailable, to facilitate patient-oriented research. These units include specialized research nurses, dietitians, biostatisticians, and professional staff and provide customized facilities including hospital rooms, metabolic kitchens, computer equipment, and sophisticated laboratories, all aimed at expediting clinical research.

THE ORIGIN OF THE GCRC MODEL

The Warren Grant Magnuson Clinical Center at the NIH campus in Bethesda opened in 1953. This 500-bed hospital is entirely devoted to clinical research. The Magnuson center has housed much of the intramural clinical research program of the NIH and has emerged as a premier training center for generations of American physician investigators. These former NIH trainees have subsequently joined the faculties of many medical schools and extended the ideals and achievements of the Magnuson center to a nationwide effort in biomedical research.

THE EXTRAMURAL CLINICAL RESEARCH PROGRAM OF THE NIH

The GCRC Program of the NIH National Center for Research Resources, initiated in 1960, supports a nationally distributed network of centers (Fig. 1) that are modeled after the Magnuson center (3). These GCRCs are usually configured as geographically discrete units within hospitals of academic medical centers. The network of GCRCs hosts multicategorical research for diseases that affect both children and adults. The centers, which are awarded on a competitive basis, are present in 59 of the nation's 127 medical schools; some institutions have more than one center. In addition, the GCRC Program funds three other centers at the Scripps Clinic and Research Foundation, the Massachusetts Institute of Technology, and the Rockefeller University. The distribution of GCRCs closely parallels the population density across the United States.

The nationwide network generally consists of about 75 GCRCs, each containing approximately eight beds. Conceptually, this is analogous to a 600-bed research-intensive hospital spread across the nation. It constitutes the extramural NIH counterpart of the Warren Grant Magnuson Clinical Center on the NIH campus in Bethesda. This arrangement provides support for physician investigators all across the country. Because the research foci of investigators differ, each GCRC's configuration and array of clinical research is unique. This network of intramural and extramural research, supported by the federal government, has placed this country in the forefront of basic and clinical research in biology and medicine.

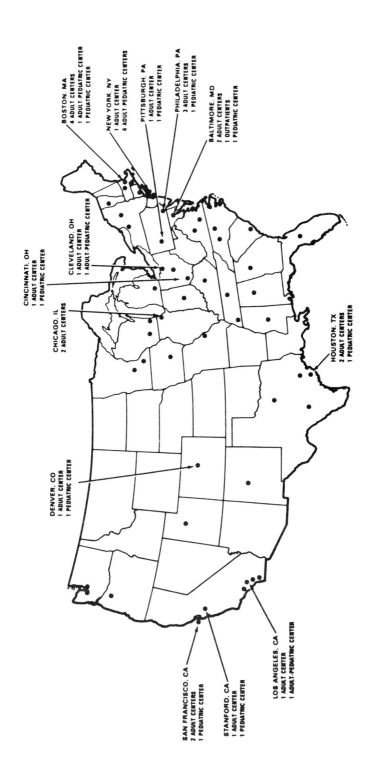

FIG. 1. Locations of the general clinical research centers. Each *dot* indicates the location of one or more GCRCs. From NIH (3).

AN OVERVIEW OF THE SCOPE OF THE GCRC PROGRAM

The GCRC program provides the clinical research infrastructure for investigators who receive their primary research support from other components of the NIH and other federal and state agencies, as well as from the private sector. Investigators who use the resources of the 30-state network of GCRCs continue to be at the forefront of biomedical research, as evidenced by the level of primary research support they receive from other NIH programs (Fig. 2) (4). In addition to the nearly $800 million in primary research support from other components of the NIH, these investigators received approximately $200 million from other federal agencies, state governments, private foundations, and industry. In 1991, 6,477 investigators carried out 4,758 research projects (4).

Research investigations mirror the research missions of the other institutes and centers of the NIH (Fig. 3) (2). The array of research conducted at GCRCs includes biotechnology, pathophysiologic investigations, clinical trials, preventive interventions, and other work. The network of GCRCs allows funneling of patients with rare diseases to units with particular expertise in those disorders. Research on AIDS continues to be a major focus, with progressively more research centering on the consequences and management of human immunovirus (HIV) infection. Undoubtedly, GCRC-based investigators will be the "trailblazers" for gene therapy of a number of diseases for which no effective therapy currently exists.

THE GOALS OF THE GCRC PROGRAM

The goals of the GCRC Program are

* to make available to medical scientists the resources that are necessary for the conduct of clinical research
* to provide an environment for studies of normal and abnormal body function and for investigations of the cause, progression, prevention, control, and cure of human disease
* to provide an optimal setting for controlled clinical investigation
* to encourage collaboration among basic and clinical scientists
* to encourage, develop, and maintain a national corps of expert clinical investigators
* to serve as an environment for training other health professionals in clinical research

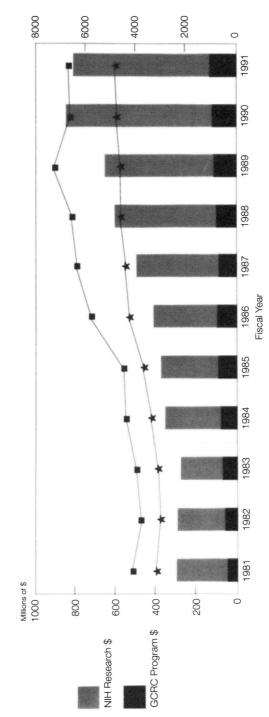

FIG. 2. Support to GCRC-based investigators and scope of the program. The *darker portion* of each *bar* indicates overall support from the GCRC Program. The *lighter ortion* of each *bar* indicates primary NIH research support to GCRC-based investigators. The *squares* indicate the number of investigators using the GCRC, and the *stars* indicate the total number of research projects conducted each fiscal year. From NIH (4).

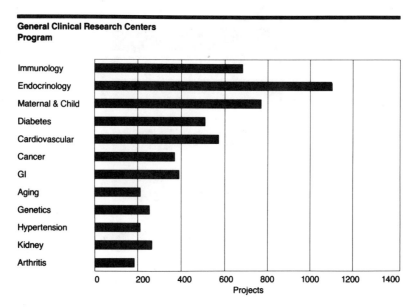

General Clinical Research Centers Program

FIG. 3. Types of research conducted at GCRCs. From NIH (2).

- to provide resources so that advances in basic knowledge may be translated into new or improved methods for patient care

WHAT IS A GCRC?

Although most centers are geographically discrete units within the setting of a university-associated hospital, they are not a fixed part of the hospital. Rather, the package of services constituting the GCRC is a renewable, competitive, NIH-supported resource designed to provide an infrastructure for high-quality clinical research. In addition to providing free room and board for study patients, the GCRC provides specialized research nurses, research dietitians, biostatisticians, computer systems managers, computer hardware and software for database management and analyses, hospital-based research ancillary costs (laboratory tests, medications), and outpatient facilities. A center constitutes an institutional resource for multidisciplinary and multicategorical research.

THE COMPONENTS OF THE GCRC

Most centers are geographically discrete and usually provide both inpatient and outpatient research facilities within the setting of a university-associated hospital. The outpatient facility may serve as a site for screening or follow-up of patients, or entire research protocols may be conducted in the outpatient area. Outpatient clinical research encompasses not only traditional outpatient visits, but also prolonged research visits of up to 10 to 14 hours. Support for off-center research beds, known as scatter beds, is also provided at many centers to accommodate research patients who require specialized facilities that are available only in other areas of the hospital—for example, in neonatal units, intensive care settings, or psychiatric units.

Centers frequently have specialized laboratories that provide routine tests in an accurate, timely, and cost-saving manner, as well as more sophisticated analyses required by at least three different investigative groups. Techniques may range from simple glucose, electrolyte, and calcium and phosphate measurements in blood and urine to stable isotope determinations, magnetic resonance spectroscopy or imaging, and viral transformation of patient cell lines for genetic studies. Metabolic kitchens are often required for studies of hypertension, metabolic bone disease, diabetes, lipoprotein abnormalities, and other disorders. These investigations may require dietary histories or special dietary manipulations. The GCRCs are staffed with specially trained research nurses and dietitians to facilitate high-quality clinical research on the centers. Timed samples of biological fluids are collected and labeled properly, a seemingly simple task that may be almost impossible at hospital sites other than the GCRC.

Most centers provide a biostatistician to assist investigators with initial study design and, subsequently, with data analysis. To complement that effort, most centers now have a computer systems manager to help investigative teams computerize data for subsequent biostatistical analyses. Software for data management and graphics production, developed under the direction of the National Center for Research Resources, has been custom-designed for patient-oriented clinical research.

The specialized personnel and other resources available at a GCRC are configured to facilitate clinical research for both the investigator and the research subject. Clinical investigators are not charged for any of the resources described.

THE ADMINISTRATION OF A GCRC

The administrative arrangement of a GCRC is shown in Fig. 4. A center constitutes an institutional resource. Because of that, the principal investigator is usually a dean at the medical school or another individual for whom administrative authority transcends departmental boundaries. The principal investigator is ultimately responsible for the GCRC and communicates guidelines from the NIH GCRC branch to the program director. The day-to-day management of a center is provided by a program director, who is an accomplished physician investigator. Associate directors assist the program director in various administrative aspects of the center—teaching and manpower development, oversight of laboratory activities, and quality of research patient care, to name but a few.

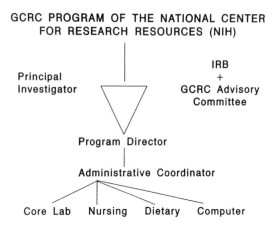

FIG. 4. Administrative management of a GCRC.

All protocols conducted at the GCRC have to be approved by the institutional review board, which evaluates risk-benefit ratios, and by the GCRC Advisory Committee, which determines scientific merit and need for the GCRC facility. The GCRC Advisory Committee categorizes and prioritizes submitted protocols, thus assisting the program director in allocating resources. For example, subjects may be categorized as Type A, pure research subjects for whom all expenses are covered; Type B, patients who require routine medical care but are also participating in a research protocol (such patients must be charged for the hospitalization); Type C, nonresearch patients who are boarders at a discrete center and must face regular hospital charges; and Type D, research subjects who are part of an industry-sponsored protocol, wherein all charges are covered by industry. The GCRC Advisory Committee also prioritizes scientific protocols in terms of scientific quality, likelihood of publishability, and need for the resources of the GCRC. In some centers, priority scores run from a rating of 1 for the best protocols to 5 for the weakest. Such scores may assist the program director in determining utilization of the unit when there is great demand.

An administrative manager assists the program director in record keeping and budgetary matters. The administrative manager has most of the responsibility for preparing an annual report to the NIH, which permits a comprehensive review of the functioning and accountability of each unit. Moreover, the administrative manager assists the program director in coordinating the various components of the GCRC to permit the smoothest, most efficient operation of the unit. In some centers, weekly chart conferences are held with all section heads. The needs of inpatients and those about to be admitted are discussed, thereby benefitting both patients and investigators.

THE CLINICAL RESEARCH PROCESS

It is a common perception that advances in clinical research go directly from the bench to the bedside. Actually, most research begins at the bedside and proceeds according to the scheme depicted in Fig. 5 (5). The physician investigator is extremely important in this entire process because it is either the astute attending physician or the clinical investigator who initially recognizes an unusual clinical problem.

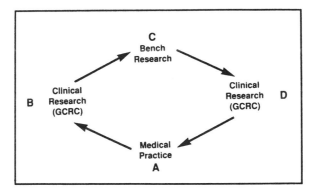

FIG. 5. Characterization of the relationship between basic and clinical research. From Vaitukaitis (5).

Let us consider an example to illustrate the clinical research process and the important role of the GCRC (Fig. 5). A doctor in practice may be confronted with several patients with kidney stones. In ordering relevant tests, the doctor may find that urinary calcium excretion is often elevated. To validate this observation, the physician investigator may wish to admit a series of kidney stone patients and age- and sex-matched normal subjects to a GCRC, where urinary calcium excretion can be measured on a constant metabolic diet. The investigator finds that a large proportion of kidney stone formers do have hypercalciuria compared to normal control subjects. Next, the investigator wishes to learn what is causing the hypercalciuria in this subset of patients. Pathophysiological tests conducted on the GCRC might include the measurement of fasting urinary calcium (a marker of bone resorption or renal calcium leak) and of the response of urinary calcium to an oral calcium load (an indirect measure of intestinal calcium absorption). Direct isotopic measurement of intestinal calcium absorption and assessment of calciotropic hormones in serum might also be performed. The investigator finds that the majority of kidney stone formers seem to have an "absorptive hypercalciuria" (i.e., normal fasting urinary calcium excretion but an increased intestinal calcium absorption). About a third of the patients have high serum calcitriol ($1,25$-$(OH)_2D$) levels, which could explain the high calcium absorption, but in most patients the increased intestinal calcium absorption is out of proportion to the normal calcitriol levels. To determine if the absorptive hypercalciuria may be related to the calcitriol levels, an agent is given which temporarily lowers calcitriol levels. This agent, which is a useful probe but not suitable for long-term use, reveals that not only the patients with high calcitriol levels, but also even some patients with normal calcitriol levels improve as calcitriol levels are reduced.

These physiological studies performed at the GCRC are analyzed, and it is determined that there are at least three types of absorptive hypercalciurias. Two of these types seem to be vitamin D-dependent due to either increased production or increased sensitivity to calcitriol. A third subset apparently has a primary gut hyperabsorption of calcium that is independent of vitamin D. Attention is now focused on the large subset of patients who seem to be vitamin D-dependent. One question is why these patients have an increased sensitivity to vitamin D. It is hypothesized that these patients may have an "up-regulation" of the $1,25$-$(OH)_2D$ receptor either in response to increased $1,25$-$(OH)_2D$ synthesis (calcitriol is known to up-regulate its receptor) or because of an inherited abundance of $1,25$-$(OH)_2D$ receptors. Further studies will be performed in the laboratory on lymphocytes and skin fibroblasts from patients and normal controls, perhaps in collaboration with nonclinical investigators with expertise in cellular and molecular biology. Scatchard analysis will be performed to determine the number and affinity characteristics of the $1,25$-$(OH)_2D$

receptors. Northern blot analysis will be used to measure mRNA coding for the calcitriol receptor. The stability of the calcitriol receptor will be assessed. Functional sequelae of the $1,25$-$(OH)_2$D-receptor interaction will be evaluated, such as inhibition of lymphocyte proliferation (by thymidine incorporation) or stimulation of the 24-hydroxylase enzyme in fibroblasts. It may also be determined whether exposure to $1,25$-$(OH)_2$D *in vitro* is associated with a greater up-regulation of $1,25$-$(OH)_2$D receptors in the cells from patients with absorptive hypercalciuria compared to normal subjects. Let us assume that, with the assistance of laboratory colleagues, the physician investigator is able to demonstrate that some patients with absorptive hypercalciuria do have an up-regulation of the $1,25$-$(OH)_2$D receptor.

Next, the physician investigator may wish to develop a safe and effective treatment for absorptive hypercalciuria. Phosphate preparations are known to inhibit calcitriol synthesis, but available preparations are rapidly released, causing cramping and diarrhea and provoking secondary hyperparathyroidism. Moreover, they are mostly sodium salts, and sodium is known to increase calcium excretion. In collaboration with a pharmaceutical company, a new slow-release, potassium salt of phosphate is developed. Once again, the problem must be taken back to the GCRC to study the pharmacokinetics of the new phosphate preparation, as well as to determine whether the new preparation will safely reduce $1,25$-$(OH)_2$D synthesis or correct the up-regulated state of the calcitriol receptor, lower intestinal calcium absorption, and restore normal urinary calcium excretion. If short-term physiological tests are promising, then the GCRC will also be essential in facilitating long-term clinical trials to test whether the new drug is safe and effective in reducing the incidence of kidney stones. Finally, if this drug is approved by the FDA, a new treatment for kidney stones may be introduced into medical practice.

THE EVOLUTION OF A GCRC RESEARCH PROJECT

As indicated in Fig 6, a clinical research project begins when an investigator gets a good idea. The idea may have been generated by recent hands-on clinical experience, by reading an article, by attending a scientific conference, or by communication with other investigators. The question being asked should be important to the investigator and to the scientific community. Search of the literature would be advisable at this point to make sure that the project has not already been accomplished. Investigators should choose projects that either they or their collaborators have the tools to explore. Creativity must be tempered with practicality. The question should be constructed as a hypothesis.

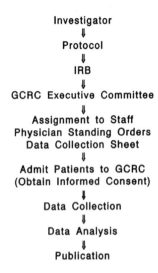

Fig. 6. Steps in the development of a research project at the GCRC.

Before the protocol is written, the researcher should discuss the project with a biostatistician, addressing important issues such as sample size, endpoints, and statistical design.

Having carefully considered the hypothesis, background, methods, and statistical design, the clinical investigator generates a protocol, which must first be considered by the IRB. This committee generally includes scientists, laymen, clergymen, ethicists, and legal counselors. The IRB must decide that the benefits to the individual and to society outweigh the risks and that all possible precautions are taken to ensure the safety of the subject being tested. The IRB must also determine that a clearly written, understandable consent form accompanies each scientific protocol so that proper informed consent can be obtained. Once approved by the IRB, the protocol can next be considered by the GCRC Executive Committee. This committee is composed of active, seasoned GCRC investigators, biostatisticians, and the administrative staff and section heads of the GCRC. Frequently, suggestions will be made to improve the scientific quality of the research proposal and to iron out any logistical problems in its implementation.

If approved by the IRB and GCRC Executive Committee, the research project may proceed. For Type A investigator-initiated studies, patients are provided free room and board, including special metabolic diets. Costs for routine medications and laboratory tests are provided.

The scenario at an optimum center might be as follows. Even before the first patient is admitted, a research nurse is assigned to the protocol and meets with the investigator to generate a standing set of physician orders, as well as appropriate data collection sheets for that particular protocol. The nursing staff performs venipunctures and assists in special procedures. Experienced research nurses may be counted on to collect timed blood, urine, and fecal samples properly and to process the samples appropriately. The nurses also assist the investigator by charting data in the flow sheet.

At the initiation of a study, during the data accumulation phase, and at the conclusion of a project, investigators are invited to present their work at weekly GCRC conferences. The GCRC Program Director and his or her associates, other GCRC staff members, and other active investigators are present to provide feedback and help avoid pitfalls. At the conclusion of the project, the facilities of the Computerized Data Management and Analysis System (CDMAS) are available to investigators. The biostatistician and systems analyst will teach the investigator to use the specially designed software to generate graphs and figures and to perform statistical analysis. The paper is now put into final form and is ready for publication, with support by the GCRC grant acknowledged.

THE TEACHING ROLE OF THE GCRC

Based on suggestions at the Program Directors' Meeting in Reston, Virginia, in December 1991, as well as on recommendations that are being advanced through the NIH strategic planning process, it has become increasingly apparent that the GCRCs should provide an institutional focus for clinical

TABLE 1. *The teaching role of the GCRC*

- Student and resident elective rotation
- Postdoctoral fellows working with established investigators
- Clinical Associate Physician (CAP) Program
- Minority Clinical Associate Physician (MCAP) Program
- Training of other health professionals (research nurses and dietitians)
- Weekly chart and data conferences
- Monthly seminar on introduction to clinical research
- Monthly seminar on practice of clinical research
- GCRC Young Clinical Investigator Award
- National symposium on techniques of patient-oriented research
- Publication of book: *Techniques in Patient-Oriented Research*

research training. Some of the ways in which the GCRC may serve as a training resource are outlined in Table 1.

One way in which GCRCs have served as a focus for clinical training is by the provision of student and resident elective rotations, in which trainees participate in all aspects of GCRC function, meet with the various section heads, and are encouraged to prepare a research protocol on a problem of their choosing. Some of these proposals have resulted in NIH grants and publications. Another well-established form of training continues to be the close relationship between postdoctoral fellows in various specialties and established investigators, who serve as mentors and role models. In my opinion, this is the most important training that occurs in the setting of the GCRC. Other health professionals such as research nurses and dietitians also receive valuable training at the GCRC. All of these individuals interact and learn from one another as well as from other GCRC personnel at chart and data conferences.

Under the 20-year-old Clinical Associate Physician (CAP) Program, each GCRC can apply for a supplemental grant to bring a young physician or dentist on board to provide the experience and knowledge that could lead to a career in research. Now the CAP program has a sister program, the MCAP (Minority Clinical Associate Physician), which is aimed specifically at young minority physicians and dentists. Under both programs, the funded center gains a valuable young worker and the young physician gains a mentor, a stimulating environment, and research experience. The CAP is generally a person who has an M.D. and has completed internship, residency, and at least 2 years of subspecialty training but does not yet have an R01 grant. During the CAP training period, such an individual gains additional research experience under the guidance of a mentor and may accumulate pilot data on a project, which may facilitate the acquisition of an independent NIH grant (R01) upon completion of the CAP. The new MCAP program differs in that a minority physician can apply either after subspecialty training or fresh out of residency. At the earlier stage, the mentor at the funded center would be allowed to have more input into the research proposal, since the applicant might not yet have had an opportunity to do research. The NIH assists MCAP applicants in finding suitable sponsors.

The CAP program funds about 15 new physician researchers each year out of about 30 applications received. The past two decades have seen more than 200 CAP recipients, most of whom have stayed in academic medicine and received their own NIH R01 grants. Clinical Associate Physician awards have benefited not only academic investigators, but also some individuals who have chosen to work in the pharmaceutical or biotechnology industries and those who have entered medical practice with a stronger scientific basis.

Recently, the GCRC at Dallas inaugurated a comprehensive training and support program for young clinical investigators. It is directed by Charles Y.

C. Pak, M.D., the principal investigator of the GCRC and the assistant dean for clinical research. The GCRC has been the focal point of the training program. The training efforts include a seminar entitled "Introduction to Clinical Research." This course comprises ten 90-minute seminars, held monthly and given by senior faculty, covering an introduction to and the definition of clinical research, conflict of interest, protocol preparation, informed consent, study design, statistical analysis, nutritional support, general laboratory techniques, molecular biological techniques, and the role of the GCRC. A second seminar, "Practice of Clinical Research," is offered to those who took the introductory course; the advanced course provides a direct "hands-on" experience in clinical research. It comprises ten 90-minute seminars held monthly and led by the same senior faculty. Materials from already completed research projects with funded research grant applications and publications are utilized for training. Although the actual topics and data chosen for this course may not be in the area of expertise or research of participants, the participants are encouraged to apply principles generated from this course to their own research area.

Another innovative program introduced in Dallas is the GCRC Young Clinical Investigator Award. From responses of participants in the above two courses, the major impediment in the initiation of a clinical research study is the lack of "seed money" for research. Without preliminary data, funding is precarious. Thus, a pilot program providing $20,000 in direct research support was inaugurated as the GCRC Young Clinical Investigator Award in the spring of 1992. To be eligible, the applicant must be a physician at the level of assistant professor who has completed the two courses on the introduction to clinical research, with a patient-oriented research project to be conducted at the GCRC, and with no other independent research support. Applications are reviewed by the GCRC Executive Committee, and the selection is based on scientific merit and the need for the center. An award is made semiannually. The source of the support, by special arrangement with the university, is a fixed fraction of royalties from drug developments (of the principal investigator) that are deposited in this account to remunerate the GCRC for partially providing the resources for drug development. There has been an enthusiastic response to this program, which represents an effective means to recruit new investigators for participation at the GCRC.

Based on successful seminars at Dallas, a nationwide symposium on techniques of patient-oriented research has been inaugurated, under the co-sponsorship of the GCRC Program of NCRR (National Center for Research Resources) and the University of Texas Southwestern Medical Center at Dallas. The symposium's overall objective is to offer training in fundamental techniques in patient-oriented research for clinical researchers to better equip them in translating exciting discoveries in the laboratory to the bedside. This annual course is intended for young physicians desirous of obtaining training, as well as for senior investigators who wish to organize a similar training program at their institutions. For further dissemination, the training seminars have been published in the form of this book.

CLINICAL RESEARCH AT THE DALLAS GCRC

The scientific productivity of the GCRC at Dallas will be highlighted as an example of a reasonably successful unit. This GCRC was funded in 1972 and opened in 1973. It consists of an 11-bed inpatient unit and an outpatient facility including three examining rooms. In its 20 years of operation, the GCRC has accommodated approximately 500 research protocols, of which 110 are currently active. The inpatient unit is typically 70% occupied, and the outpatient area sees 400 patients per month. In a typical year, 25 original articles in major peer-reviewed journals, 16 chapters and reviews, and 23 abstracts for presentation at national research meetings are generated.

Some of the recent scientific accomplishments of the Dallas GCRC are as follows. Progress has been made on a safe and effective treatment for osteoporosis utilizing intermittent, slow-release sodium fluoride. A new reflection ultrasound instrument was developed to measure bone quality and strength noninvasively *in vivo*. Three drugs have been formulated, tested, and given FDA approval for the treatment of kidney stones, and three additional drugs are in the early stages of development. The initial report describing the ability of lymphomas to cause hypercalcemia by excessive calcitriol production has been confirmed in numerous laboratories. Evidence is being sought that absorptive hypercalciuria and idiopathic osteoporosis may represent milder forms of calcitriol excess or sensitivity.

The Dallas GCRC has had a long interest in lipoprotein metabolism, starting with the Nobel Prize-winning work of Goldstein and Brown in discovering the LDL receptor pathway and the related lipoprotein clearance studies of Bilheimer and Grundy. The early investigation of hepatic hydroxymethylglutaryl coenzyme A (HMG CoA) reductase inhibitors, including Mevacor (Lovastatin), was performed in Dallas. Particular attention has been paid to the role of diet and drugs in controlling plasma lipids, and the benefits of a high-monounsaturated-fat (olive oil) diet have been revealed. The role of dietary micronutrients with antioxidant properties such as ascorbate, alpha-tocopherol, and beta-carotene in preventing LDL oxidation and hence atherosclerosis has been reported.

Evidence has been accumulated that susceptibility to diabetic complications may be related to the activity of the aldose reductase pathway. A multicenter trial was initiated which has provided strong evidence that oral administration of ursodeoxycholic acid improves symptoms, liver function tests, and liver histology in patients with primary biliary cirrhosis. Several new muscle enzyme disorders in patients from around the world have been described and treated. A novel therapeutic approach to rheumatoid arthritis that targets endothelial cell surface adhesion receptors (monoclonal antibodies against ICAM-1 receptor) and prevents recruitment of leukocytes into inflammatory extravascular sites has been initiated.

All of these exciting developments have occurred at just one GCRC. It is necessary to multiply these achievements 75-fold to begin to grasp the contributions being made by the GCRC program nationwide to the overall clinical research effort.

CLOSING THOUGHTS

As the former director of the National Institutes of Health's GCRC Program and current director of NCRR, Judith Vaitukaitis has had the unique opportunity to observe the forefront of clinical research carried out across this country. Her appraisal of clinical research is very realistic: "Nothing is more demanding, more difficult, more frustrating, more time-consuming, and requiring more creativity than clinical research. On the other hand, nothing is more gratifying than the fruits of clinical research that allow the clinical investigator to not only define the cause of a disease but also to develop novel therapies to alleviate or even cure a disease" (5).

Another thoughtful observer of the biomedical research scene is Daniel E. Koshland, Jr., editor of *Science.* He noted that

the line between pure research and practical application has always been difficult to draw. Some like to claim they are doing pure research with no practical purpose in mind. There is an implication that "pure" is not only nobler but also more difficult intellectually than "applied" research. Equally vociferous are those on the applied side who suggest that they labor for the good of mankind, whereas the ivory tower types are simply enjoying themselves. Those demarcations are gone forever, or should be. It is a wise person who can state with certainty what basic research result will never be practical, or what applied research will not lead to new basic insights, or which is intellectually more demanding (1).

There are different kinds of clinical research. Those attracted to the type of patient-oriented clinical research conducted at GCRCs are generally more interested in studying human beings than experimental animals, in whole organisms rather than isolated cells or molecules, taking an integrative rather than a separative approach to science. Recently, there has been a perception that patient-oriented research has lagged behind basic laboratory research. The GCRC could serve an important function in helping to produce an improved balance between laboratory and clinical research. Progress in biomedical research requires a complementary and interactive relationship between basic laboratory investigation and studies in human beings. In the final analysis, only through clinical research are advances in basic science ever translated into advances in human health.

ACKNOWLEDGMENTS

This work was supported by NIH Grants PO1-AM-20543 and MO1-RR-00633. The author thanks Ms. Betty Bousselot for expert secretarial support.

REFERENCES

1. Koshland, D.E., Jr. (1991): Frontiers in biotechnology. *Science* 252:1593.
2. National Institutes of Health (1990): *Program Highlights 1990*. NIH Publ. No. 91-2309 (December). National Center for Research Resources, Washington, DC.
3. National Institutes of Health (1991): *General Clinical Research Centers: A Research Resources Directory*. NIH Publ. No. 91-1433 (January). National Center for Research Resources, Washington, DC.
4. National Institutes of Health (1991): *Program Highlights 1991*. NIH Publ. No. 92-2309 (December). National Center for Research Resources, Washington, DC.
5. Vaitukaitis, J.L. (1991): The future of clinical research. *Clin. Res.* 39:145–156.

10

How to Write a Scientific Paper

Scott M. Grundy, M.D., Ph.D.

Center for Human Nutrition, University of Texas Southwestern Medical Center at Dallas, Dallas, Texas 75235-9052

Writing a scientific paper that describes one's research findings is the essential last step of the research process. Unless an investigator completes this step and publishes the result, the research itself is largely a meaningless effort. Therefore, learning to write a research paper should be an integral part of the education of any investigator. Although the principles of scientific writing are similar for all of the sciences, certain elements must be emphasized for the clinical investigator.

There are several textbooks on how to write good scientific articles, and each presents its unique insights. I have been particularly influenced by the text by Dr. Peter Woodford entitled *Scientific Writing for Graduate Students* (Woodford, 1968). Dr. Woodford was a colleague of mine at the Rockefeller University in the 1960s. We both worked under the leadership of Professor E. H. Ahrens, Jr., who is a prominent clinical investigator; Dr. Ahrens has taken a great interest in the teaching of scientific writing to his students. This chapter reflects my training under Drs. Ahrens and Woodford, but it also expands on my own experience gained as an independent investigator. In this chapter, I will attempt to identify some of the principal questions that must be dealt with by *junior clinical investigators as they attempt to bring their research projects to fruition and to publish their findings.*

WHO SHOULD BE THE AUTHORS?

Many scientific papers have multiple authors, and the order in which the authors sign the paper generally is deemed to be of some importance. The first name on the paper usually is reserved for the person who actually performs the experiments and brings the study to completion. Frequently, this person is the junior investigator. The last name in sequence customarily is reserved for the "senior" author, that is, the head of the laboratory under whose guidance the work has been performed. The senior author typically provides the other authors with the general idea for the particular project and usually governs the funds and other resources used in the undertaking. In the educational role, the senior author characteristically works with the first author on the preparation of the final manuscript, more than do other coworkers. Other authors as a rule are collaborators, and frequently they add key ingredients to the project. The order of their names on the publication usually is ranked according to the relative importance of their contribution to the overall study.

The names of the authors on a paper and even the order of names can become a contentious issue, and hard feelings can result if the issue is not dealt with in a forthright manner. For this reason, the role of each participant and the order of names on a manuscript ideally should be determined before the study actually begins. Young investigators tend to be disinclined to bring the matter up with their senior investigator, who, in turn, often is careless about it. However, since the potential first author generally has the most to gain by being named the first author, it behooves this person to confront the matter head on and to bring the senior investigator to a decision at the beginning. This is especially so if the paper is to have multiple authors. A frank dialogue at the beginning of a study can preclude much heartache later.

In bench-type research, in contrast to clinical investigation, multiple studies often are carried out simultaneously, and it may be difficult to foresee what will be the final results or what form a publication may take. Thus, predetermination of the sequence of authors' names may not be possible. In clinical investigation, in contrast, the delineation of authors, including the order of names for specific projects, more often is less difficult. A protocol normally must be approved by an institutional review board, and the preparation of the protocol for this board is helpful for defining the relative roles of the various individuals participating in the project. This fact will help to determine ahead of time the order of names on a manuscript.

WHEN IS THE RIGHT TIME TO PUBLISH?

When young investigators are involved in research they are always faced with the query of when they have acquired enough new data to write a research paper. A common aphorism in the academic world states "publish or perish." This rule holds more truth than most of us would like to admit. If a young faculty member fails to publish research papers, there will be no promotion and no new grant funds. Two reasons frequently underlie failure to publish. One is the attempt to publish one's research too soon—before the study has reached maturity; this can lead to rejection of papers and to discouragement. The other reason is the failure to bring work to completion. In general, research is done step by step; it transpires by quantum jumps rather than as a continuous progress. A key step in the development of a flourishing research program is the ability to recognize what constitutes a "publishable unit" of research. The right time to publish a paper is when one such unit has been completed.

A researcher must cultivate the ability to think in terms of incremental steps of progress. Publication will be greatly simplified if the researcher can visualize the essential contents of a paper before the research is started. One way to do this is to establish an experimental design (or protocol) that will constitute a completed study. The clinical investigator usually is required to submit a protocol to the institutional review board before starting a study, and this exercise usually preestablishes what will constitute a full study. Thus, when the protocol has been executed and the data analyzed, the time has come to begin writing the paper.

Some researchers unfortunately fail to write their papers within a sensible period after completion of the study. After the data are collected they can languish in notebooks and remain neglected for far too long. Failure to bring a completed study promptly into a publishable form has several drawbacks. For instance, a paper may lose its timeliness, and its contents can be superseded by the publication of other work. Thus, both priority and relevance are lost. Dereliction in bringing one's project to finish often impedes the undertaking of new ventures. Failure to complete a manuscript has a way of draining zeal and enthusiasm away from an investigator. It is basically the responsibility of the first author to take the lead in writing the first draft of the manuscript, and failure to do so constitutes an injustice to collaborators who have invested of their time and effort in the project. Thus, while one should avoid premature publication, failure to prepare a manuscript in a reasonable period often results in an assortment of undesirable consequences.

One important point to make about clinical investigation is that negative results can be as valuable as a positive outcome. Because of limited data in human research in general, most carefully controlled investigations are worthy of publication. Young investigators thus should make it a rule to strive to publish their results, even if the results do not fully live up to expectations. The completion and submission of a manuscript, even one of limited consequence, will be an important learning experience. Certainly the first few papers of a young investigator generally are not of the quality of those of a mature researcher, but the process of writing and publishing must begin somewhere. A final point is worth making: research that does not seem important at the time it is published may later take on significance and meaning that were not foreseen.

THE ESSENTIAL HYPOTHESIS

Research in general should be "hypothesis driven." This is to say that the investigator should develop an hypothesis that is the foundation of the experimental design. One way to formulate an hypothesis is to pose a question of dispute. As a rule one can say that the more profound the question, the greater will be the implications of the results. Young investigators frequently have difficulty in articulating consequential and well-defined questions. The hypothesis should be specific and circumscribed in scope. It should address a particular issue. Ideally, the hypothesis to be tested is set forth as precisely as possible at the beginning of the study, in the development of the protocol and experimental design. If the hypothesis is sound, and if it leads to a focused study, this will go a long way toward making the final paper less difficult to write, to say nothing about betterment of its overall quality.

In general the best approach is to address only one question per study. This will make the paper less complicated to write and easier to read. Papers that address multiple questions often end up mixing conclusive results with dubious findings, and the final product is a confused amalgam that is strenuous and even perplexing to read, much less to comprehend. If multiple questions are being set forth in a single study, it often is better to recognize this at the beginning of the project and to divide the project into several segments. For instance, three short papers with clear-cut findings are easier to read than one long paper in which all observations must be presented and discussed together. Longer papers that contain dissimilar and unconnected information are especially troublesome. Experience has shown that the prospects of getting a paper accepted are better if the paper is relatively short and contains a single principal discovery.

THE SINGLE MOST IMPORTANT FINDING OF THE STUDY

A critical first step in writing a paper is to determine what is the single most important finding of the study. The whole paper should be written around this finding. The principal finding should be given the highest priority both in the presentation of the results and in the discussion of its import. Exposition of other results at the same time tends to dilute the key message of the paper. If possible, additional findings should be presented in a way that underscores the most conspicuous discovery of the investigation. Secondary findings should bolster the primary result and not obscure it. Therefore, before beginning the written exposition, the authors need to set forth in a few sentences the essential discovery of the inquiry. This conclusion can guide the development of the manuscript and should be the underpinning of the entire manuscript.

WHAT IS THE MOST SUITABLE JOURNAL?

The choice of a journal in which to publish a research paper can be based on several criteria. The journal should be as eminent as possible, and it should reach an audience that will give the greatest attention to the article. Preferably, the journal chosen will have a wide dissemination. Some journals, such as the *New England Journal of Medicine,* the *Journal of the American Medical Association,* and the *Journal of Clinical Investigation* are relatively general, and all three reach a large audience. The former two are directed toward the whole medical community, whereas the latter is read principally by clinical researchers. In addition, there are a large number of specialty journals that tend to be read only by specialists (e.g., gastroenterologists, diabetologists, cardiologists). In the minds of many people, the more general journals carry a greater prestige, but this apparent advantage usually is only temporary. In the long run, it is the quality of the manuscript that counts, and the paper will be remembered more by its contents than by the journal in which it was published. There are many examples of very famous papers published in relatively obscure journals. Nonetheless, the perceived quality of the journal must be one factor affecting the decision about where to submit.

Other factors also can be taken into consideration when choosing a journal. Rapidity of publication is one. If a journal normally takes 1 year to publish from the date of submission, it is less tempting to try than one that takes only 6 months. On the other hand, it is often better to publish in a prestigious journal even if it takes somewhat longer in reviewing and processing. Finally, articles require a high quality of photographic reproduction, and this may be provided by only certain journals.

As a general rule, an investigator should submit his or her paper to the best and most reputable journal available, provided that there is a chance for publication. It is often difficult to predict at the time of submission whether a paper will be accepted. Acceptance depends to some extent on the luck of the draw (i.e., who reviews the paper). Some reviewers are tough and critical, whereas others are lenient and sympathetic. Editors tend to accept reviewers' recommendations, and if one or two reviewers are negative about the paper it will have little chance of acceptance. Quality, of course, is the prime factor determining acceptability, but fortune plays its role. For this reason, if a paper is rejected, the authors should adopt a philosophical outlook. If the paper is of reasonably high quality, one should take a chance on the best possible journal. Courage is often rewarded by acceptance and, even if the paper is rejected, the reviewers may provide valuable comments that will assist in revision for submission of the manuscript elsewhere.

A note of caution nonetheless must be introduced at this juncture. Junior investigators often overestimate the quality of their initial investigations. Their ardor for their project may cause them to assess its results at a higher quality than it genuinely deserves. A result often is the desire to submit the manuscript to one of the more renowned journals. The senior investigator may have to introduce a moderating influence. It is no disgrace to have a paper rejected, but neither is it prudent to waste time on a hopeless prospect. Still, even senior investigators do not have crystal balls, and their judgment may not be inviolate. The best solution to the quandary of where to publish is to have a candid discussion of the possibilities and to choose accordingly. Senior investigators are inclined to appreciate the weaknesses of a study, whereas more junior researchers tend to see only its strengths; in most cases the journal of first choice probably should represent a compromise between these extremes of assessment. In any case, the first submission should not be to the journal of last resort; instead it should go to the most prestigious journal in which there is a reasonable chance for acceptance.

IN WHAT ORDER SHOULD THE PAPER BE WRITTEN?

The way not to write a scientific paper is to start at the beginning and to write sequentially all the way through. This approach is not practical. A suggested alternate approach is presented in Table 1. According to this master plan, the tables and figures should be constructed first. In so doing, it will be learned whether there are enough data to constitute a full paper. Certainly, appropriate statistical analysis will be required in construction of the figures and tables. A word of caution, however. One should not have the figures prepared in final form on glossy prints at this early stage. The final art work and printing should be done only when the rest of the paper is complete. Often there will be changes in the figures right up to the final day.

In general, the first part of the text to draft should be the methods section. Next will come the results section. These two sections are the heart of the paper. One can then write the introduction and discussion, in that order. If the discussion is written before the introduction, there will be a propensity to overlap the two. If the introduction is written first, the discussion can be an extension of it, and it can concentrate more on the current findings. It is often useful to write the text of the introduction and the discussion without references; citation of the literature can be added later after several revisions of the text. Of course, when citations are added, the text may have to be altered to be consistent with the references. The next step is to construct a title for the paper, and, finally, the abstract is written. For practical reasons, the references, title, and abstract need not be written until the body of the text has gone through several drafts.

TABLE 1. *Master plan*

1. Construct tables and figures
2. Write methods section
3. Write results section
4. Write introduction
5. Write discussion
6. Add references
7. Construct title
8. Write abstract
9. Finishing touches

THE OUTLINE OF THE MANUSCRIPT

Writing a paper can be aided greatly by formulating an outline ahead of time. An outline will assist in the organization and design of the paper and will help to give it balance. Preparation of an outline exacts thought, and one must attempt to visualize the whole of the manuscript at the beginning. There are several approaches to generating an outline. For example, while the study is in progress key points can be stored on cards, and when the study is finished these can be categorized as the first step in an outline. Next, one can prepare a topic outline, listing the essential elements of the paper in a logical order. Finally, the topic outline can be expanded to include key sentences under each topic. Unfortunately, most authors do not approach the scripting of papers so systematically. Instead, they begin to draft whatever comes into mind, with no idea of how the whole section will read when finished. This is particularly true of the introduction and discussion sections. To a large extent the arrangement of the methods and results sections is determined by the procedures and data, but the introduction and discussion sections are more open ended. Therefore, it is useful principally to make outlines of these latter two sections.

TABLES AND FIGURES

Data can be presented in either of two ways (i.e., as tables or figures). Depending on the type of data, one or the other of these means of presentation may be preferable. For example, tables are chiefly useful for presenting quantitative data, whereas figures often are better for showing a qualitative picture. The use of tables can expedite the presentation of statistical information. On the other hand, figures can be used to amplify numerical data. Perhaps the greatest advantage of figures is that they have more visual impact than do tables. Figures make a greater immediate impression than do tables but, over the long haul, the numerical data contained in tables often grow in value. One of the dangers of using figures is that they are more "subjective" than tables. Figures often are drawn in a way to convey the authors' prejudices about what the data show. They typically are constructed to make a point, and if they bestow a distorted picture, the reader will be misled. A good rule is to give tables priority for the major part of the data display and to reserve figures for amplification of the information contained in the tables.

Several features of the construction of tables are worthy of consideration. Tables should be as uncomplicated as possible, and they should contain only key data. If it is necessary to present a large volume of data, multiple tables should be used. It is better to have multiple modest tables than one or two complex listings that are laborious to read. Simple tables typically are more demanding to construct than are expansive ones; effort is required to condense data, and the decision to eliminate nonessential results often is exceedingly hard to make. Most investigators are reluctant to withhold or discard data that were obtained through long and arduous labor, but for the sake of intelligibility and clarity this may be imperative.

One question that always arises about clinical investigation is whether to present individual data or only to show group means. Sometimes the reviewers or editors will prefer one or the other. One reason to show individual data is to allow the reader to search for findings that may not have been noted by the authors. If readers are intensely interested in the results of a paper, they may want to scrutinize the primary data and to draw their own personal conclusions. Indeed, a reader may choose to reanalyze the data by a different procedure from that presented, and this can only be done if the primary data are available. Still, inclusion of primary data on individual subjects requires additional space, often with marginal additional information for the general reader, and the editor may not allow it. The exhibition of excessive primary data, moreover, may cloud or obscure the principal findings of the paper. The reader may not be able to see the forest for the trees if too much attention is given to the trees.

The procedure of multiple revisions of tables will improve and enrich their quality, and with the availability of word processors we are blessed with the opportunity to make revisions rapidly and with a minimum of exertion. Columns and lines can be moved about with the greatest of facility, and the final outcome should have all of the attributes of a high-quality table. Since tables and figures are the heart of the manuscript, the extra time needed to bring them to the highest possible quality is time well spent. This endeavor will significantly strengthen the chances that the paper will be accepted. Papers should be and generally are accepted on the quality of their data; if the data are presented in a clear and concise fashion, chances for acceptance are improved.

Figures are useful for showing curves that plot one parameter against another (e.g., time versus activity). Such information is inconvenient although not necessarily impossible to show in tables. Equations for curves with correlation coefficients can be presented in tables, but a more lasting impression can often be achieved with figures. If there is a large number of correlations to be shown, the key data can be displayed in figures, and secondary findings (e.g., multiple correlation coefficients) can be given in tables. Figures are especially suitable for exhibiting certain types of primary data (such as instrumental tracings, electrophoresis patterns, and photomicrographs); data of this type cannot be demonstrated easily in tables.

If figures are used, certain general principles should be followed about their construction. Since their size will be reduced in the journal, the graphs and lettering should be large enough to read easily after this reduction. If this rule is followed, the lettering may look too large in the original graph, but after reduction it will appear to be the right size. As mentioned above for tables, extra time spent in the preparation of the figures undeniably will increase the probability that the paper will be accepted. A few key figures can make or break a paper in the eyes of the reviewers. Further, the quality of the legends is important; to the extent possible, a figure should stand on its own. Legends ought to contain enough information to guide the reader to the key features of the figures. In first drafts of the paper, it is better to err on the side of putting too much information into the legend. Later, this can be condensed to the right length. In many publications, the legends contain insufficient information to enable the reader to understand fully the information contained in the figure. The author obviously will completely grasp the meaning of the figure without the legend, but the assumption should not be made that the reader will be able to do so. The legend is an important guide to discrimination of the key elements of a graph.

THE METHODS SECTION

The Description of the Patients

If the manuscript contains clinical research, the methods section usually will include a description of the patients. Unfortunately, it is common for papers on clinical investigation to present inadequate description of the participants in the study. One often gets the feeling that the authors were trying to obscure information about their patients, possibly because of excessive heterogeneity in selection. This may not be the case, however, and the authors may merely be careless in presentation. The essential features of the patients— age range, sex, body weight or body mass indexes, and primary clinical features—should be included in the description. Such other characteristics as smoking habits, medications, and level of physical activity may be helpful to the reader. Often a table that catalogs the essential attributes of the study population will facilitate and streamline the description. At some point in this section, it is important to indicate that the investigation was approved by the appropriate institutional review board.

The Experimental Design

Many clinical papers exhibit a relatively poor description of the experimental design. Perhaps the authors believe that the design of the study is self-evident from the other material in the methods and results sections. This, however, is not always the case. Thus, a separate subsection called "Experimental Design" should be added to the methods section. Often the description of the design can be simplified by adding a figure containing the key elements of the protocol. In most clinical investigations, the protocol has been carefully described in the application to the institutional review board. The experimental design section of this application may be helpful in writing the same section in the final manuscript.

If the experimental design involves changes in dietary intakes, the composition of the diet should be described in detail. It is common to describe the diet of investigational patients inadequately. The percentages of fat, carbohydrate, and protein should be listed. It may be useful to give the average caloric intake if this information is available. Intakes of micronutrients and vitamins should be listed. If the diet compares different types of fat, the fatty acid composition of the dietary fat should be given. If the authors have any information on dietary assessment (i.e., how the composition of the baseline diet or therapy diets was determined), such information will be useful to the reader.

Analytical and Clinical Procedures

The methodologic procedures used in the investigation should be described sufficiently to allow them to be repeated by other workers, either from the text or after referral to original sources. If the methods taken from the literature are modified, a full description of the modification is needed. An important component of the methods section is the presentation of the statistical methods employed to analyze the data. Most investigators would do well to consult with a biostatistician before starting a clinical project. Unfortunately, consultation often is sought after the study is over, and consequently the quality of the analysis frequently is compromised.

THE RESULTS SECTION

For most papers, the results section can be relatively short. This section is essentially a description of the tables and figures and a guide to them. One can expand on what is not in the legends. Two common mistakes are made in the results section. One is to put information in the results that should be in the methods section, and the other is to incorporate discussion and speculation, which rightly belong in the discussion section. For example, a description of baseline characteristics of a group of patients normally should go under "Methods." Moreover, if the experimental design is clearly delineated under "Methods," it will not be necessary to explain the design under "Results." Further, the authors should resist the temptation to interpret the results of their study in the results section. Interpretation and speculation belong to the discussion section. Finally, one should avoid repeating the information in the tables and figures in the text of the results. Certainly, the actual values listed in the tables should not appear in the text, except for emphasis. On the other hand, the text may be used to give percentage changes between two sets of numerical data that have been presented in tabular form.

THE DISCUSSION SECTION

Without question the discussion section is the most difficult part of the text to write for the inexperienced investigator. One can more easily learn the rules for writing the methods and results sections. A good discussion section, however, requires not only that one has a reliable understanding of what the experimental data actually mean but also that one has the ability to communicate in writing the essence of this meaning. The current results further must be put into the perspective of the whole literature of the topic under investigation. A sound discussion section should be well balanced and should avoid overstatement of the significance of the findings. Furthermore, it ought to give a fair assessment of the existing literature as it relates to the current results. It is discourteous to other researchers not to give full credit to data that contributed to the current hypothesis. On the other hand, if one does not adequately discuss and convey the significance of the current findings, one does a injustice to one's own work. Since a high-quality discussion section is so difficult to write, the investigator should spend extra time in writing and reworking it.

In spite of the difficulties involved in writing a discussion section, some investigators believe that this section is the least important part of the paper.

This is because the primary purpose of the publication is to convey the essential data of the study and, to some workers, the authors' own interpretations of these findings are largely irrelevant. It may be true that in the long run the primary data assume increasing importance at the expense of interpretation. Over a period of years, with advances in the field, explanations within a given field change, and an author's own view of the measurements assumes less importance. Nonetheless, when the paper is written, the author may have given more thought to the topic under investigation than has anyone else, and undoubtedly the author may have more insight into the meaning of the results than do other investigators. The discussion section thus provides the author with an opportunity to express a unique view of the significance of the research.

Perhaps the most important thing the authors can do in the discussion section is to state unequivocally the most important finding of the paper. The hypothesis outlined in the introduction often sets the stage for this purpose. Did the result confirm or refute the primary hypothesis? If the experiment was designed appropriately to test the hypothesis under analysis, then the single most important result probably will connect to the hypothesis. Still, studies often reveal results that are radically unexpected, and the most important finding may be utterly unrelated to the hypothesis under examination. For most studies this will not be the case, but discovery of the unforeseen has been the basis of the greatest advances in science. Thus, all scientific studies are not limited to being hypothesis-testing enterprises. Regardless, near the beginning of the discussion section, the authors should state explicitly the single most important finding of the study.

Beyond the single most important finding, most papers will have additional results that must be reviewed. To the extent possible, secondary findings should be considered in the light of the major observation. If the discussion section deals with a large number of separate issues, it probably will be disjointed and difficult to read. The effort accordingly must be made to weave all the findings of the paper into an integrated whole. Secondary findings should have a supporting role; each cannot convincingly stand on its own as a separate issue of discussion. There is the temptation to consider and speculate about different constituents of the database. If possible, this snare should be avoided; if it is not, the whole discussion section will be impoverished.

Two fundamental questions can be asked about every paper: (a) what is important? and (b) what is new? The matter of how to address "what is important?" was considered above. The question of "what is new?" deserves equal attention. If the chief discovery of the paper is not new, this may lessen its importance in the eyes of many readers. Of course, one must be careful in claiming priority of discovery. Many editors will not allow direct claims of priority and, in any case, it is prudent to indicate the priority of one's discoveries in an oblique way. One way to do this is to note that the current results are a meaningful addition to previous reports. The limitations of preceding accounts can be explicitly noted, and just how the current findings move the field forward certainly can be set forth. Thus, whereas direct claims of priority are in poor taste and may lead to unnecessary friction with other authors, there are usually ample opportunities in the discussion section to stake one's claim to priority in an indirect way.

Although every investigator would prefer to make innovative observations, confirmatory findings can be of substantial worth. Frequently, the authenticity of new claims will remain in doubt until they have been confirmed. Take, for example, the recent claim of "fusion in the kitchen." If it had turned out to be true that fusion of hydrogen can be accomplished by simple chemical procedures, the implications for future energy supplies would be enormous. Unfortunately, the assertion could not be substantiated by other investigators, and the failure to attain confirmation was of extreme importance to the whole field. Likewise, in clinical investigation, confirmatory studies hold a place of special consequence because initial studies usually are not definitive. Thus, in writing a discussion section, attention should be given not only to what is new, but also to what is confirmatory. One need not apologize for introducing confirmatory data, but instead one should denote it with clarity. Likewise, if a previous finding cannot be verified, this too should be pointed out. Since papers often overstate the significance and generalizability of their contents, restoration of perspective by failure to affirm prior results can provide a valuable service to the field.

An appropriate review of the literature in the discussion section is critical. The current results should be put into perspective of the existing field of knowledge. It is unfair to ignore previous research that has either influenced the present study or provided meaning to it. The ability to integrate what is known from the past with what was found in the current work requires experience and perspective, but it is indispensable for the creation of a well-rounded discussion section. Of course, the number of potential articles that might be cited is immense, and a careful selection of the most germane and pertinent articles is necessary. Citation of the literature can be expedited by having key articles at hand during the writing of the discussion. This will help to assure that the articles are quoted correctly. In a hurry to complete manuscripts, some writers refer to original sources from the quotes of other papers. To do this does not serve the interests of the original authors, and the writer is obliged to reread the original paper before quoting it. Other workers in the same field naturally are sensitive when reading a manuscript from a "competitor" and, if their previous research has not been quoted accurately or quoted at all, resentment, indignation, and even bitterness may result. Certainly it may not be possible to quote all pertinent literature, and it is difficult to satisfy or please all other workers in a particular field. Nonetheless, authors should be sensitive to this potential problem, and every effort should be made to be fair and honorable when referring to the literature. Still, one must not forget that the purpose of writing the discussion section is to bring the current findings into perspective; it is not to adulate and flatter prior investigators. Good judgment thus is required to set current and previous research into balance without demeaning what went before.

Authors would be wise to foresee possible criticisms of the reviewers and to explicitly indicate the major limitations of their study. This strategy often will defuse or soften censure and thereby will strengthen the possibility that the paper will be accepted. The exercise of defining the boundaries and defects of one's investigation may at the same time disclose its strengths. Such will not only assist the author in writing a more measured discussion section, but it also may elevate the quality of the study in the eyes of the reviewer. Science demands that those who aspire to uncover its secrets maintain a degree of modesty, and forthright acknowledgment of limitations often will mute the criticism of reviewers.

Out of the limitations of a study may grow new questions for future research. The reader should be given insights on how the current study may lead the field in new directions. Such speculation may give the reader new perspectives into the implications of the current findings. The old saying that many discoveries raise more questions than they answer often is true, and, unless these questions are well articulated, the discussion section will be incomplete. Authors, of course, should be selective in their speculation about future research. To the extent possible the logical next step in research should be pointed out, and one should resist the temptation to engage in "wild speculation." Research papers not only must impart new knowledge, but also should open up new areas of investigation. Some readers of papers will readily see the implications of new findings, but the authors can use the opportunity of the report to provide guidance to other investigators for future research.

Finally, the discussion section should have a concluding paragraph. This paragraph can take various forms depending on the message the authors want to leave with the readers. It can recapitulate the essential conclusions of the study. It can indicate the major implications of the findings, or it can point out what new avenues of investigation may be opened up by the report. There is no need to restate what is in the abstract and discussion, but at the end the reader should be left with the essence of the paper. The authors should take advantage of the closing to convey to the reader the most important information contained in the paper. Therefore, the authors need to give extra time and thought to the concluding paragraph.

THE ABSTRACT

The abstract is the last part of the text to be prepared. Several comments can be made about its contents. A brief statement of the problem under investigation is needed. This can be followed by an indication of the hypothesis to be tested. The abstract should not launch immediately into the results of the study but should outline for the readers the reasons behind the investigation. This introduction can be followed by a brief description of the methods used in the project. The research findings come next. The authors should attempt to provide key quantitative data; the findings ought not to be described merely in qualitative terms. Actual data will considerably improve the quality of the abstract. If the single most important finding of the paper can be presented in quantitative terms, so much the better. Finally, the major finding should be summarized in the conclusion of the abstract. A good abstract will stand on its own. No reference needs be given to what will be discussed or presented in the body of the paper. Since abstracts are often reproduced separately from the paper itself, the authors need to be aware that for many readers their only contact with the paper will come through the abstract. The authors therefore should take advantage of this opportunity to create the best possible abstract, literally, a very short version of the paper. The preparation of an appropriate abstract takes time; it is not just a last minute operation before the paper is completed and submitted.

THE TITLE

The last item of the text is the title. It is common practice to quickly jot down the first title that comes to mind. A better way is to make a list of five or six possible titles and to consider each meticulously. The title should be discussed among the coauthors, and modifications need to be made until the best possible title has been defined. In general, it is better not to use titles that ask a question or make a declarative statement. The latter in particular should be avoided; such titles impose a conclusion on the reader before the study has been read. The reader may not agree with the interpretation and, moreover, declarative sentences restrict the range of possible interpretations that can be applied to the investigation. Vague and general titles (e.g., "Effects of . . . ") likewise are not desirable, especially if a more specific description of the substance of the study can be developed. The titles of papers, of course, go in an author's bibliography, and they will be read by those who are evaluating one's scientific accomplishments. In addition, titles are given in *Current Contents* and similar publications, and they may determine whether a particular reader will take the trouble to find and read the article. In this sense, the title is an advertisement for the article. All of these reasons justify taking the additional time required to prepare the best possible title.

THE REFERENCES

General comments about review of the literature were presented under "The Discussion Section." In preparation of the citation list, it is important to check the journal requirements for the reference format. Journals vary in their formats for references, and there is no single acceptable arrangement. Further, just keeping the numbers straight between the text and citation list is not always simple. Right before submission of the manuscript, it is helpful to read the reference numbers out loud and to compare them with their placement in the text. This preferably should be done with a coauthor or secretary; two people are more likely to pick up mistakes than one. Carefully check the spelling of names of the authors; one must not forget that the one name misspelled will probably be the major reviewer of the manuscript. To prepare for future publications, investigators would do well to develop a reference list with a computerized reference organizer. Several software programs currently are available for this purpose, and they can be extremely helpful in the organization and retrieval of references.

SUGGESTIONS FOR WRITING MANUSCRIPTS

Learning to write manuscripts of high quality can only come through the process of writing. Of course, writing scientific papers requires the basic skills of writing in general, and if these have not been acquired in school they must be learned later. If one has problems with writing effectively, it may be worthwhile to seek the assistance of a tutor. Several excellent textbooks also are available to guide one in the improvement of writing skills. A word of caution is in order. Young investigators probably should not pay too much attention to the writing habits of their mentors or to the style found in most scientific journals. In many cases these are not of high quality.

The general rules for writing obviously pertain to scientific writing. One should strive to be as simple and concise as possible. Every sentence should be reread carefully, and the meaning of every word examined. Unnecessary words must be eliminated, and a conscious effort should be made to shorten sentences wherever possible. Sentences are more effective when they are written in the active voice; also, try to use verbs instead of nouns where feasible. One should seek out noun clusters and stacked modifiers, and attempt to break them up. Remember the true adage: the adjective kills the noun! Authors need to be aware that there are now computer programs that will scan a text and make suggestions for improvement of grammar. Junior investigators may find these to be helpful.

Multiple revisions are the key to good manuscripts. In my experience, the schedule shown in Table 2 represents an effective approach for writing a manuscript. The availability of word processors greatly facilitates the revision of manuscripts. If one follows the schedule outlined in Table 2, a good reworked draft, but not final product, should result at the end of one week. The next steps in the preparation of a paper are outlined in Table 3. As indicated, a reworked draft can be prepared in one week. It is better to put the paper away for another week to clear away the mind's blind spots for the manuscript's weaknesses. The process used in the first week can then be repeated in the third week, and the manuscript can be brought to a state of completion. As a rule, one should not submit a manuscript on Friday afternoon; instead, it should be read over one more time during the weekend. A few small mistakes are always found in the final reading. Then the paper can be submitted early the next week.

DEALING WITH REVIEWERS' COMMENTS

For all investigators, whether junior or senior, a first reading of the comments of reviewers and editors is traumatic. One's hard work frequently is roundly criticized. The following suggests one author's approach to coping

TABLE 2. *Schedule for rewriting*

Day of week	Day	Night
Saturday	Write first draft	Go to movies
Sunday	Write first draft	Complete first draft
Monday	Put into computer	Rework draft
Tuesday	Put into computer	Rework draft
Wednesday	Put into computer	Rework draft
Thursday	Put into computer	Rework draft
Friday	Put into computer	Read a book

TABLE 3. *Completing a manuscript*

Week 1:	Prepare a reworked draft
Week 2:	Put paper away for one week
Week 3:	Complete the manuscript
	Don't submit the paper on Friday afternoon.
	Reread the paper over the weekend.
	Submit the paper during the first part of the week

with the trauma of reviewers' comments. Upon receiving the decision letter and comments, this author reads the letter and comments through at once. They always produce an unpleasant emotional reaction, but all temptation is resisted to write a nasty letter to the editor or to complain to other investigators. The paper then is put away for a week or two and is forgotten. Thereafter, when the comments are reread, they usually are not so bad after all and often are quite helpful. In fact, they usually reveal significant weaknesses in the paper that need attention. It is best not to take the comments personally or even too seriously and to handle them with dispatch. The paper should be completed as soon as reasonable thereafter. If perchance the paper is rejected, the same process is followed. The only difference is that instead of returning the revision to the same journal, it is submitted to another. Only after an article has been rejected by three or four journals should one give up on it. It is my experience that ultimate rejection of a manuscript is rare.

SUMMARY

The writing of a scientific paper is like any other skill; it requires a good grounding in the fundamentals, and perfection comes only with repeated efforts over a long period. Nonetheless, good scientific writing is to a large extent a learned skill, and the points outlined in this paper may provide shortcuts to learning the hard way. The ability to compose a manuscript is of little value if the research project and its results are not meaningful, and one's primary efforts should go into carrying out the project. Nonetheless, if a good project is not brought to completion, which means writing and publishing a manuscript, it will be of little or no value to the field. Thus, learning to write a good scientific paper is an essential part of learning to do high-quality research, and without this skill one cannot achieve the status of an independent investigator. The publication of papers represents the link between prior and future investigation, and unless previous research is brought into press it will not be possible to move ahead to further work. The writing of good papers requires a great deal of time and effort, and one must be committed to this critical step in the research process to achieve success. The suggestions set forth in this manuscript are made in an effort to facilitate this pivotal exercise.

REFERENCE

Woodford, F.P. (1968): *Scientific Writing for Graduate Students: A Manual on the Teaching of Scientific Writing.* Rockefeller University Press, New York.

Index

Index